THE
21-DAY
SUGAR
DETOX
DAILY GUIDE

New York Times bestselling author
Diane Sanfilippo

Victory Belt Publishing
Las Vegas

First Published in 2018 by Victory Belt Publishing Inc.

ISBN-13: 978-1-628602-70-8

Cover design, photos, & recipe photos by Diane Sanfiippo
Cover and interior portraits by Charlotte Dupont
Interior design by Yordan Terziev and Boryana Yordanova

Printed in Canada

TC 0521

CONTENTS

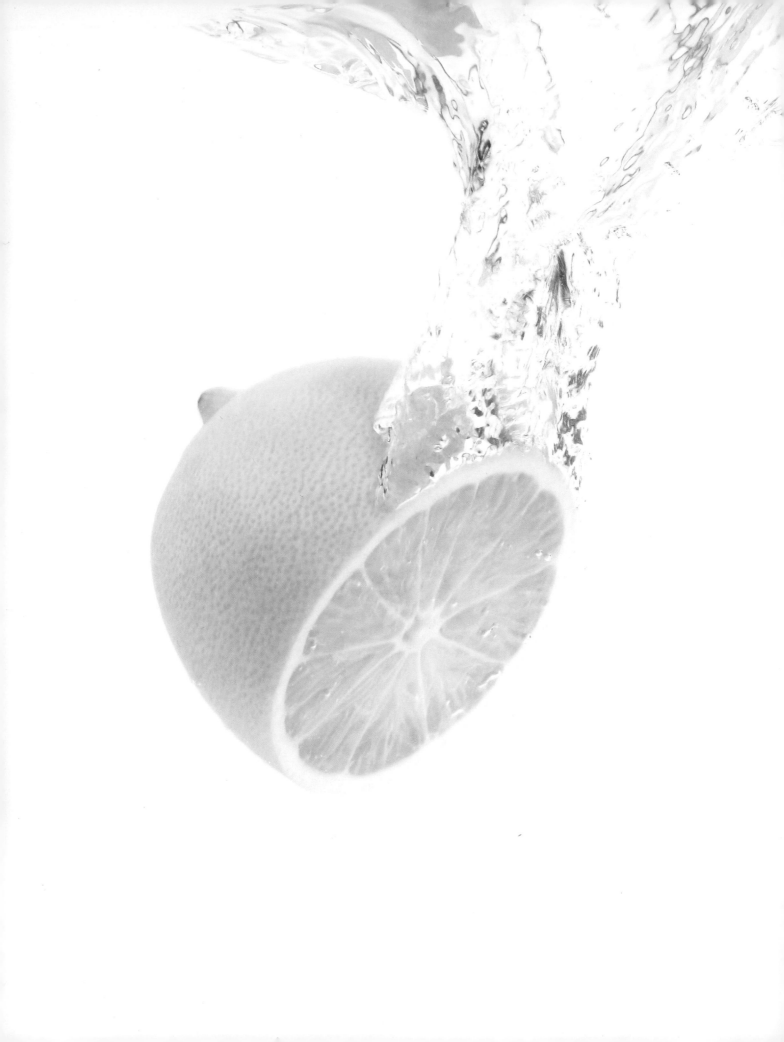

INTRODUCTION

When I was growing up, I was the Candy Girl. If I earned two dollars for completing some chores, you can bet that every penny of it was going to be spent on Snickers, Rolos, Three Musketeers, Blow Pops, Tootsie Rolls, and Jolly Ranchers. And this relationship with sugar and sweets didn't end with my youth. Nope, it followed me well into adulthood, when I had free rein to eat whatever I wanted, whenever I wanted. Birthday cake for breakfast? Yes, please! Leftover pie for an afternoon snack? You better believe it. It wasn't just sweets, either—I loved sugar in any form. I'm talking about refined carbs that turn to sugar in your body, like bagels, pretzels, bread, and pasta.

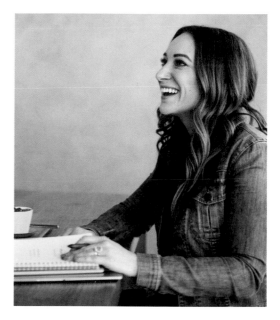

When I decided to lose weight after college, I dove headfirst into dieting. If it was a processed "health" food, I ate it: high-fiber cereal, soy cheese, low-fat granola bars, and non-fat anything. I'd eat meals that left me feeling full for maybe two hours and then reach for snacks to prop up my energy level and keep me from zombie-level hunger.

Now, there's a difference between getting hungry as you naturally should and getting to that "hangry" (hungry + angry) place because you've overdone it on bad carbs and your blood sugar jumped up only to come crashing back down. I never knew that it was possible to get hungry without also getting shaky, feeling like I was going to pass out, sweating, or even feeling nauseated, like I would do anything to get my hands on something to eat. I knew I was on a blood sugar roller coaster, but I didn't know how to get off it!

Eventually I learned that eating meals that were more balanced—with adequate protein and plenty of fat, as well as veggies—could help me feel better. I resisted at first, because I was convinced that eating fat would make me fat. Boy, was I wrong. When I finally decided to stop being afraid of fat and give this new approach a shot, I ate a reasonably sized meal of chicken thighs and kale cooked in some coconut oil, and I wasn't hungry again for several hours. And when I got hungry, I just got hungry. I was finally able to eat a meal and feel satisfied.

What a difference protein and fat can make! Once I cut out sugar, refined foods, and gluten, my blood sugar stabilized. It was like a miracle. I could go out with plans to be gone for over an hour and not have to jam a snack into my purse—food freedom!

After a year of gloriously even blood sugar levels, I had a slipup. It was around four in the afternoon, and I had worked through lunch and was hungry—*really* hungry. And instead of taking myself home to eat, I stopped at the candy store. The Candy Girl had been dormant for many years, but she hadn't quite been obliterated yet! I bought a quarter pound of gummy candies, licorice, and other assorted super-sugary goodies, and I ate the entire bag. At once. About an hour later, it hit me. My massive sugar intake led to the hardest blood sugar crash I'd ever felt. I was right back to that full-blown hangry place—shaking, sweating, and feeling like I was going to pass out. I actually felt like I might fall to the floor. Once I finally started to feel better, I knew without a doubt that my dietary changes had been the right way to go—and I was never going to do that to my body again.

Removing sugar and refined foods from my diet has given me the energy I always knew I should have, improved the quality of my sleep, and even helped to alleviate the chronic sinus infections I struggled with for many years. It's amazing what can happen when we give our bodies what they want, rather than simply what's readily available.

As a result of my own blood sugar roller coaster experiences, years of holistic nutritional studies, and then more years of working with clients as a nutrition consultant and teacher, I developed the 21-Day Sugar Detox. I wanted to help people get off the blood sugar roller coaster and give them a way to jump-start the process of kicking those sugar and carb cravings.

What Is the 21-Day Sugar Detox?

At its core, the 21-Day Sugar Detox (21DSD) is a three-week real-food-based program that helps you bust sugar and carb cravings naturally. There are no required supplements, shakes, pills, or powders. I originally created this program in April 2010, and it has since helped hundreds of thousands of people to live healthier, happier lives, free from the chains that sugar once had on them.

The best part about this program is that it's not about deprivation or dieting! On the 21DSD, you'll eat plenty of healthy whole foods that nourish your body. Rather than going hungry and feeling like you need to struggle or power through the program, you'll eat whenever you're hungry, using the tons of delicious, healthy recipes right here in this book and beyond.

Why Try the 21-Day Sugar Detox?

There are four main reasons to follow the 21DSD:

1. Regulate blood sugar levels and lose body fat.

By changing the food you're eating for three weeks, you'll regulate your blood sugar levels and kick-start the physiological process that encourages healthy fat loss. The nutrient-dense whole foods you'll be eating will provide your body with the vitamin- and mineral-rich calories it needs for the countless functions it carries out on a daily basis, giving you more energy than you previously had.

2. Quell your sugar cravings.

When you begin eating differently every day, you start to crave the new foods you're eating. It sounds a little crazy, but I've seen it happen time and time again with our detoxers—they go from craving a morning pastry to waking up excited for eggs, bacon, and kale!

Avoiding refined foods, sweeteners, and even super-sweet whole foods lets all of the beautiful, naturally sweet foods truly taste sweet again. And, in turn, sugary processed foods become cloyingly sweet to your reset palate. You'll enjoy the wonderful and natural sweetness of a green apple in a whole new way and with a new appreciation after completing the 21DSD.

3. Reduce inflammation in your body.

Inflammation is the body's response to a problem. When your body thinks there's a constant problem, it lives in a chronic state of inflammation. This steady, low-level, systemic inflammatory state is at the root of just about every chronic disease imaginable.

Sugar consumption plays a role in chronic inflammation in two main ways:

1) Depleted nutrient stores from overconsumption of bad carbs lead to a chronic state of stress in the body.

2) Chronically high and/or low blood sugar—the blood sugar roller coaster, which comes from consistently ingesting too many bad carbs—creates a stress state for the body.

But the 21DSD doesn't just eliminate sweeteners and sugary processed foods; it also eliminates some of the most common food allergens: gluten, soy, corn, and (for some) dairy. This program gives your body a period of relief from the irritation and systemic inflammation that can be caused by these foods. For example, when you reintroduce gluten or soy after the twenty-one days, you may discover that they're problematic for you, but you'd never have known that without eliminating them completely for three weeks.

The list of physical symptoms that can result from the combination of dysregulated blood sugar and the consumption of foods your individual body doesn't tolerate includes but is not limited to:

SHORT-TERM POTENTIAL EFFECTS

- Acne, rashes
- Fatigue
- Mood swings
- Muscle fatigue or weakness
- Other food addictions
- Premenstrual syndrome (PMS), painful periods
- Susceptibility to colds and flu
- Unrestful sleep

LONG-TERM POTENTIAL EFFECTS

- Adrenal fatigue or dysfunction
- Alzheimer's disease
- Anemia
- Cystic acne, eczema, psoriasis
- Depression, anxiety
- Insomnia
- Insulin resistance, type 2 diabetes
- Myelopathy, neuropathy
- Polycystic ovary syndrome (PCOS), infertility
- Substance abuse

When you focus on eating real, whole foods and eliminate not only processed and refined foods but also common allergens and irritants, the positive effects can be staggering.

4. Create new, healthy habits.

There's a good chance you came to this program because it can teach you about what to eat to feel your best, to avoid that 3 p.m. slump at the office (and the subsequent trip to the candy jar), and to break the chains sugar and carbs have had on you.

But I hope that you also learn how to navigate a healthy lifestyle beyond your twenty-one days. This program will raise your level of awareness about where sugar hides and how it impacts you and your body *personally*. While this book will carry you through the detox day-by-day, you are not going to move through the program exactly the same way as anyone else. You are unique in many ways—from your lifestyle to your habits to your tastes—and your experience on the program will help you figure out how you like to form new habits and what works best for you in adopting new lifestyle changes, so that you can continue your new way of eating after the twenty-one days.

You'll also learn something about yourself! You'll learn that you *are* capable of doing hard things, that you *can* learn new skills, and that you can feel happy and content in choosing to cook and eat healthy foods. Since you'll likely be eating lots of new-to-you foods and eliminating foods you're used to eating, this program will help you to learn a whole new way to look at food, from shopping at the grocery store and cooking food at home to choosing from a menu and building your plate to balance your energy throughout the day. The habits and skills you'll learn on the program can be carried through to your life beyond the 21DSD.

> "Give a man a fish and he eats for a day. Teach a man to fish and he eats for a lifetime."

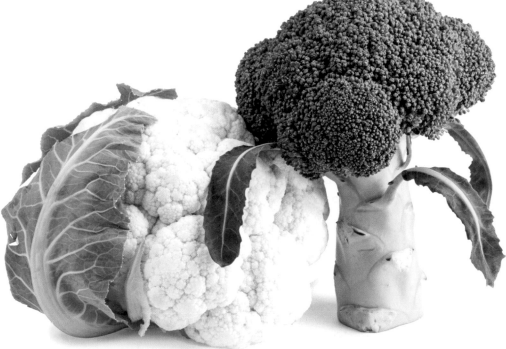

Why 21 Days?

I first designed the 21-Day Sugar Detox to last twenty-one days because research showed that it takes that long to create a new habit. However, it turns out that it takes *at least* twenty-one days to create a habit—and twenty-one is not the be-all, end-all number. We now know that, on average, it takes much longer to *fully* form a new habit—more like sixty-six days. For some it may take less time, perhaps eighteen days, and for others much, much longer, perhaps more than eight months.*

What constitutes a habit? Simple: it's something that you do on a regular basis without thinking much about it. A habit is formed when an action becomes a part of your regular activities and you don't need to concentrate or exert effort to do it.

So, if the average amount of time it takes to form a habit is sixty-six days, why keep this program to twenty-one days instead? Well, for starters, twenty-one days is a lot more manageable for most folks, and I'd be lying if I said I didn't want as many people as possible to give this program a try. That's because I know *for sure* that everyone who endeavors to complete a 21DSD learns a lot! Whether it's simply how to shop and cook better, how to order when dining out, how to read nutrition labels to find hidden sugars, or how they'd previously been set up for failure when it comes to creating healthy habits—there are countless lessons to be learned by completing a 21DSD. I don't want to turn someone away at the door, so to speak, by presenting a program that requires a commitment of more than two months.

Three weeks is also enough time to face important challenges. During your detox, it's important to encounter situations that can be challenging for your new way of eating, to help you learn how to navigate them once your 21DSD has ended even if you're not completely cutting out sugar afterward, you'll want to hang on to your new healthy-eating habits. These situations include:

- grocery shopping and cooking in a new way
- bringing food to eat at work (and storing and heating it there)
- attending a catered office meeting, where you have to navigate the offered food or avoid it altogether
- dining out with coworkers or having work meetings over meals or drinks
- dining out with family or friends (some of whom may be unsupportive)
- eating while traveling
- attending parties or celebrations

Over the course of three weeks, you're bound to encounter one or more of these scenarios. So, while I could easily extend this detox program to cover more time, I don't believe that it's necessary in order for you to learn a lot and decide how you'd like to carry what you learn into your life after your detox.

---

* Phillippa Lally, Cornelia H. M. van Jaarsveld, Henry W. W. Potts, and Jane Wardle, "How Are Habits Formed: Modelling Habit Formation in the Real World," European Journal of Social Psychology 40, no. 6 (October 2010): 998–1009.

What About After the 21 Days?

The 21DSD requires that you abide by its rules for the entirety of the twenty-one days, but not beyond that.

Since this program will carry you through twenty-one days (thirty-five if you complete the pre- and post-detox weeks), you'll be well on your way to creating new habits to bring into your everyday life after it ends. That being said, you will continue to develop and solidify your new healthy habits *after* the detox.

Here's the good news: research shows that in the span of time during which you *fully* form your new habits (remember, anywhere from eighteen days to eight months!), missing one opportunity to perform the habit didn't affect the resulting habit formation. So the big relief here is that when you take your new way of eating beyond twenty-one days, an "off" decision here or there does not a habit break!

Your success on this program will be in direct correlation with how much you believe you are in control of your own life and your own choices.

So take heart! There is great value in committing to the rules of the 21-Day Sugar Detox while you are completing the program, but afterward, strict adherence to specific rules or rigid daily habits isn't necessary for the benefits to remain. I'm most invested in your long-term success in creating healthy habits around food, not just whether you complete the 21-Day Sugar Detox. Aren't you?!

What Does It Mean to "Detox"?

When folks make a statement about "going on a social media detox," no one bats an eye. Everyone knows that the detoxer is taking a break from an activity that has deleterious effects for them. But for some reason, if you flip the script to "going on a sugar detox," suddenly folks get up in arms:

You don't need to detox from sugar, it isn't a drug.

You don't need to detox, your body detoxes naturally.

Why would you do that? Sugar isn't a toxin.

If you look up "detox" in the dictionary, you'll see that there are two separate entries: it's both a verb (short for "detoxify") that means "to remove a harmful substance," and a noun that means "a regimen intended to remove toxins from the body."

Many detractors focus on the verb and point out that our liver naturally detoxifies our body, without our changing anything about our diet. While this is true, it's not the whole story. The 21-Day Sugar Detox addresses "detox" both as a noun—by providing a program to help you break free from sugar—*and* as a verb, by helping your liver do its job.

Yes, one of the main functions of the liver is to filter impurities from the bloodstream. When we talk about whether or not we "need to detox," we're not talking about turning this process on—our liver is already detoxifying our bloodstream. But is it working optimally? Is it fully supported in carrying out its functions? Not likely. The foods we encourage you to eat on the 21DSD are specifically chosen to meet the liver's nutritional needs and support it as it detoxifies the bloodstream.

I like what the word "detox" implies about the reality of what it means to detox from sugar. Sure, sometimes it makes people feel like this program will be gimmicky (it isn't), or loaded with powders or pills you need to buy (nope), or that you'll be drinking only juices and starving for three weeks (you won't). But more often than not, calling it a "detox" opens people's eyes to the fact that, yes, sugar *is* something we can all benefit from removing from our lives, at least for a period of time.

> Detoxing can be both a lifestyle change and a physiological process. The 21-Day Sugar Detox helps with both.

Do we really need to detox from *sugar*?

While it's often stated anecdotally that sugar is as addictive as narcotics, I'm certainly not here to put something that we can safely eat in the same category as a controlled substance. While both sugar and narcotics make the reward center in our brain light up, the implications for short- and long-term mental and emotional health are *not* the same.

Furthermore, while research shows that consuming sweet foods can have mood-altering effects and may seem to help us handle stress, depression, pain, or discomfort, just like narcotics, sweets have far less severe psychological and behavioral effects than drugs. Consuming foods that are high in sugar doesn't result in a change in behavioral disposition or induce an abnormal mental state. So, though the cravings-inducing effects of sugar may be comparable in many ways to those of narcotics, they are certainly *not* the same, and calling this a "sugar detox" is not meant to imply that they are.

That being said, sugar does have a strong hold on us.* We are wired by nature to seek sweet foods—they give us a jolt of dopamine, a neurotransmitter associated with feelings of reward and pleasure. We'll talk more about dopamine and sugar on page 34, but for now, suffice to say, our bodies are primed to seek more and more sweet foods, and that's a problem today, when sweet foods are usually empty of nutrients and sugar is everywhere.

Sugar is highly available in our modern food landscape. In fact, I'd argue that the biggest reason why detoxing from sugar can be so difficult is its sheer abundance. It's hard to avoid and so very easy to get! Avoiding sugar requires effort, planning, thought, and, frankly, that you go against the way that society (and the big food companies) has designed the entire structure of eating in everyday life.

This is why the 21-Day Sugar Detox works. It's not just about ridding your body of toxins, although that certainly will happen. It's also about practicing a new way of eating that avoids the sugary cycle.

IS THE 21DSD THE SAME AS GENERAL LIVER DETOX SUPPORT?

Not exactly. While the 21DSD will absolutely support the liver in the detoxification process by supplying it with necessary nutrients, if you think you may be suffering from toxin overload (from heavy metals, environmental toxins, hormonal overload, etc.), there are additional protocols, supplements, and lifestyle factors involved with supporting liver detox. Talk with a naturopathic doctor, functional medicine doctor, or other holistic health practitioner one-on-one if you feel that you'd benefit from additional support.

---

* Serge H. Ahmed, Karine Guillem, and Youna Vandaele, "Sugar Addiction: Pushing the Drug-Sugar Analogy to the Limit," *Current Opinion in Clinical Nutrition and Metabolic Care* 16, no. 4 (July 2013): 434–439.

HOW—AND WHY—TO USE THIS BOOK

The 21-Day Sugar Detox Daily Guide is a simplified approach to the 21DSD program, broken down day-by-day. To quote Al Pacino in *Scent of a Woman*, "All information will be given on a need-to-know basis."

I first created the 21DSD in April 2010 as an online program, followed soon thereafter by a print guidebook, *The 21-Day Sugar Detox*, and its companion cookbook, *The 21-Day Sugar Detox Cookbook*. Both printed books include twenty-one-day meal plans, and together they offer more than two hundred recipes. The guidebook also includes a short day-by-day account of what to expect while on the program, as well as a Daily Success Log template, which became the inspiration for this book.

We also have an amazing online program, available at 21DSD.com, which complements all of the books for those who love accessing content from anywhere, via any device. The 21-Day Sugar Detox Online Program includes the program rules PDF, daily support videos, optional daily detox emails, and a growing community of Certified 21DSD Coaches and participants.

So with all these other options, why offer this daily guide, too? Because changing the food you eat means changing the way you think, plan, prepare, and live, and I want to support you in that process beyond simply offering rules and recipes. I want to empower you as much as possible, and also offer a hand wherever I can.

Over the years, I've listened to participants' feedback about what would help them—what would help *you*—to complete the 21DSD even more easily. I also noticed how people interacted with the materials I'd already created and drew some conclusions about what was most helpful and what else might be useful.

- Guidance for the period just before and just after the actual twenty-one days, with support and details for how to ease into and out of the detox

- Helpful details about what you're experiencing, presented in a time-sensitive way, to help you understand that you're not alone in the challenges you're facing and give you more insight about what's happening when it's most relevant to you

- Less pre-detox reading, which can feel overwhelming!

- Daily notes and mindset tips to coach you through the program

- Tips and tricks for making each day a bit easier (from me as well as from Certified 21DSD Coaches and others who've completed the program)

- Preparation checklist items for each day

- Specifics on how much to eat based on your lifestyle, activity level, and goals

- Quick-fix meals, so each day doesn't include too many recipes that require a full-on kitchen takeover

- Shopping lists for the recipes you'll be making

- Even more recipes!

The 21-Day Sugar Detox Daily Guide was born out of exactly those needs!

This book is your go-to handbook, preparation guide, FAQ resource, meal plan, simplified cookbook, and journal for the 21-Day Sugar Detox program, all in one. It doesn't replace the original guidebook or cookbook—they hold tons of information on the program and recipes that you won't find in this book. But this book can be your one-stop shop, so to speak, if you want daily guidance.

How to Use This Book

I've organized this book into easy-to-follow daily breakdowns. Start with this introduction and the program guidelines starting on page 17, then move on to the daily pages. You'll begin using the daily guide content a week before your detox begins, continue through your full twenty-one days on the detox, and finish up the week after your detox. The pre- and post-detox weeks have some good information and are there to set you up for success leading into and out of the program.

You can read just the current day's entry, read a few days ahead, or read as far ahead as you like. Then you can review each day as you are experiencing it. So, for example, you may decide to preview all of the pre-detox week by reading through all of those daily pages before you dive in, but you'll go right back to 7 Days Pre-Detox when you're a week away from starting your 21DSD and stay focused on that day's lesson, tips, and checklist. You are welcome to read ahead at any time, but I recommend you stay focused on each day as it comes along on your program so that you can tackle it before moving on.

The Yes/No Foods List (pages 19–21) and "Building Your 21DSD Plate" (pages 22–23) are the foundations of this program. The rules of the 21DSD are simply to eat foods from the Yes list and avoid foods from the No list, according to the level at which you are completing the program. There are three program levels, all designed to support you based on your current dietary profile. Level 1 is the most inclusive, Level 2 is more moderate, and Level 3 has the most dietary restrictions.

"Building Your 21DSD Plate" is your guide to figuring out portion size and assembling meals and snacks while on the program. If you are not following the meal plan in this book, no sweat! You can simply build meals and snacks using foods on the Yes list and in portions according to guidelines on pages 22 to 23.

The meal plan (pages 115–121) not only has you covered for each day's meals but also has make-ahead and make-over recipes all planned out for you within your daily prep work. I'm taking the guesswork out of what to do with leftovers, and I'll teach you how to cook ahead by keeping recipe remixes in mind even beyond your detox! Use the prep instructions during your pre-detox week, then use the shopping lists to buy your groceries each week. You'll be able to eat multiple times from each cooking session. You'll see that the meal plan has notes for what you will "cook," "make ahead," and "save" each day. While you don't have to follow the exact meal plan I've created in order to complete the 21DSD successfully, I know you'll enjoy being on the same page (literally!) with others on the detox if you decide to do so.

To track your progress in a meaningful way, I've included space for you to journal. Time and time again, 21DSD participants have told me that they wished they'd kept track of how they felt during the detox and all the small wins they made along the way. With the journal pages and prompts from each day, you'll be able to track challenging moments and learn what works best for you to overcome them. Some of what you'll track is simple data, like what you ate for each meal (especially important if you decide not to follow the meal plan) and whether you drank lots of water or had your piece of included fruit, while the rest is your area to assess yourself and how you're feeling.

Getting Started

Before you dive into the 21DSD, there are a few steps that can help prepare you for success.

Step 1: Read and review the Official 21-Day Sugar Detox Program Guidelines.

Now that you've read the introduction, review the Official Program Guidelines starting on page 17 to discover which foods you'll be eating while on the program. Then take the quiz on page 18 to determine your level, and review the portion size options on pages 22 to 23 to determine what is appropriate for you while on your 21DSD.

Step 2: Enlist support.

This is the perfect time to enlist a friend, coworker, or family member to join you on this journey. While we've got an amazing social network, including Team 21DSD, Certified 21DSD Coaches, and other detoxers, it's always easier when people around you are going through the program, too.

And if, upon reading what this program entails, you're feeling overwhelmed and think that you really want one-on-one support from a real person, we've got your back! There are Certified 21DSD Coaches around the world who can help, whether in person or online—or both! Our Certified Coaches all go through a training program specifically for the 21DSD so they can guide you through this program with the best possible support *and* a personal touch. There are coaches who specialize in working with people with particular concerns, from athletes to pregnant or breastfeeding moms to people with food allergies and autoimmunity. Our coaches have all completed the program themselves, so they know exactly what it's like to be in your shoes and can give you that helping hand when you need it. You can find a coach at 21daysugardetox.com.

While many successfully complete this program without the additional help that a coach can provide, you know yourself better than we do, and if having the support of someone you can check in with regularly will help you succeed, then by all means, sign up with a coach. Our coaches are truly a phenomenal group of practitioners who are there to support you.

> ### DETOX *HARDER*?
>
> Remember, making this program stricter doesn't mean your detox will be more successful! In fact, eating less food in general or eating less carbohydrate than you need may backfire on you and cause your detox process to go poorly. So follow the guidelines! If you are allergic or intolerant to some of the Yes foods, then of course omit them, but beyond that, stick to what the program details for you.

Step 3: Read the pre-detox days (pages 32 to 40) the week before you begin.

While you can dive into the full 21DSD right away, I don't recommend that. Lack of preparation is the number one reason why folks don't finish the program. Yes, it's a tough program, but it's far, far easier when you prepare for it.

That means following the pre-detox daily pages in this book (pages 32 to 40) for seven days before you start your 21DSD. These days will walk you through familiarizing yourself with the program, cleaning out your pantry and refilling it with detox-friendly ingredients, logging what you eat so you can anticipate what you'll need to change on the program, and more. These prep days will make everything much easier and smoother once you start your detox.

Step 4: Commit—and let the world know!

Hop on over to 21dsd.com/join to let me know that you're in! We'll ask you about your "why" and help you connect with our community. And if you think daily videos and emails would help you stay on track, this is the time to sign up for those as well through the online program. If you enjoy using social media, share one of our fun "shareable" graphics to your accounts using #21DSD so we can follow along on your journey.

Step 5: Start your 21DSD!

That's it! Once you've finished the pre-detox week, you're ready to begin with day 1 of the 21DSD. Start with the guide for that day on page 44.

> ### FIND US ON SOCIAL MEDIA!
>
> OFFICIAL HASHTAG:
> **#21DSD**
>
> RELATED HASHTAGS:
> **#21DSDrecipe, #21DSDcoach, #21daysugardetox**
>
> Instagram:
> **@21daysugardetox**
>
> Facebook:
> **facebook.com/21daysugardetox**
>
> Pinterest:
> **pinterest.com/21daysugardetox**
>
> Twitter:
> **twitter.com/21daysugardetox**

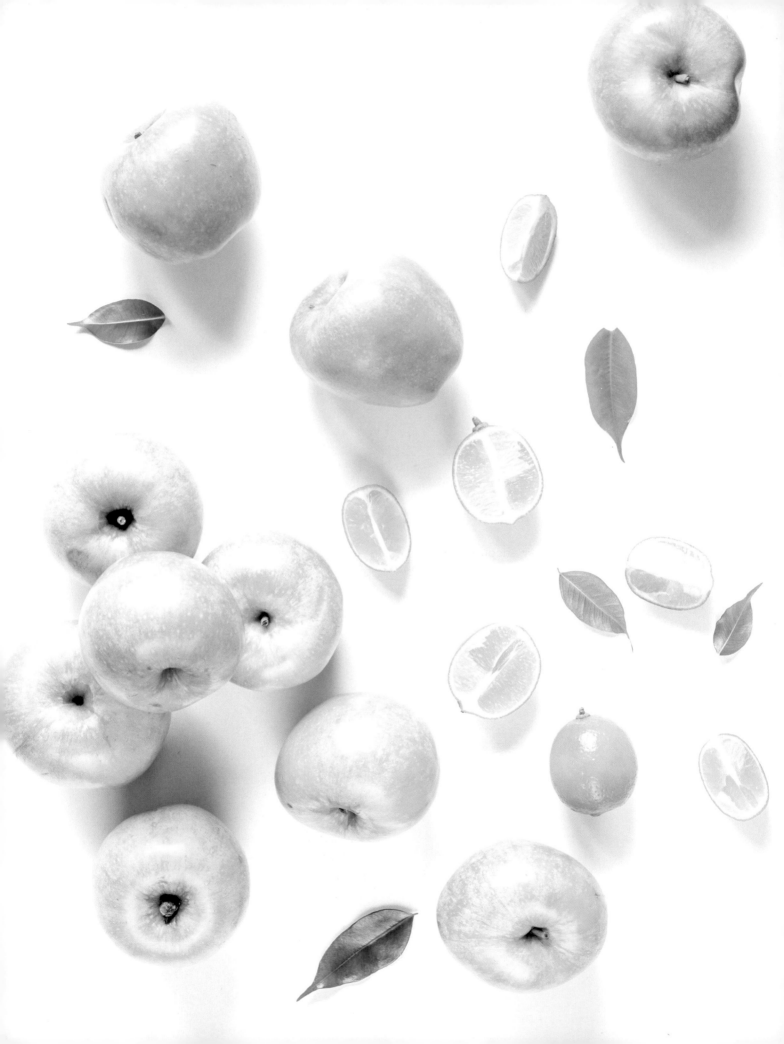

THE 21-DAY SUGAR DETOX
OFFICIAL PROGRAM GUIDELINES

In its simplest form, the 21-Day Sugar Detox can be completed by eating Yes foods and eliminating No foods (and ingredients). Some Yes foods should be consumed in limited portions, but for most, you can eat as much as you like.

Once you review the Yes/No Foods List (pages 19–21), read through "Finding Your Level" (page 18) and "Building Your 21DSD Meals" (pages 22–23). This will help you to determine how strict your program will be and your starting point for portion size. After you start the 21DSD, if you find that you need to adjust your meals based on how you're feeling, "Building Your 21DSD Meals" can help with that, too.

Is It a "Yes" Food?

While on your 21DSD, you may encounter foods that are not on the Yes/No Foods List, or you may be slightly confused about whether a particular food is included in or excluded from the program. Follow the basic principles of the 21DSD, outlined below, to direct your choices and help you figure out whether or not you should eat the food in question.

- Added sweeteners are not allowed. The only way to enjoy a somewhat sweet taste is to use the included fruits in the limited portions as outlined in your Yes/No Foods List. If an added sweetener is included in the ingredients list of a packaged item you want to eat (see the Guide to Hidden Sugars on page 109 to find hidden sweeteners), the food is not allowed. Note that some Yes foods, such as full-fat dairy on Levels 1 and 2, contain natural sugars, and these are okay.

- If it tastes sweet and it isn't included on the Yes foods list, it's not allowed. Some herbal teas taste sweet naturally, and these are allowed. If an item tastes sweet and you aren't sure about it, leave it out.

- Grain flours are not allowed. This means you will not eat any foods made from whole-grain or refined-grain flours (wheat, spelt, and quinoa flours, for example). The only flours allowed are those made from nuts, seeds, coconut, or some limited starches (like tapioca flour when used as a thickening agent in sauces).

- When in doubt, leave it out. If you find it difficult to make a judgment call about a particular food on your own, connect with us online at 21DSD.com or via social media to ask your question and get more answers and support.

Finding Your Level

For your best experience on the 21DSD program, you'll want to customize your approach based how much of a change the program will be for you, how active you are, and how strong your cravings currently are. There are three levels to the program, with Levels 1 and 2 allowing some foods that are off-limits on Level 3.

To determine the right level for you at the beginning of your 21DSD journey, circle the most appropriate responses below:

1. *Are you new to the 21-Day Sugar Detox?*

A. Yes.

B. No, I have completed it once before.

C. No, I have completed it two or more times before.

2. *I currently eat*

A. bread, pasta, and other foods made from whole grains or grain flours (wheat, teff, spelt, kamut, rye, etc.).

B. bread, pasta, and other foods made from gluten-free grain flours.

C. a grain-free, Paleo, or primal type of diet.

3. *I currently eat*

A. low-fat or fat-free dairy products.

B. full-fat dairy products.

C. no dairy products.

4. *I currently eat*

A. sweeteners or foods made with sweeteners multiple times per day and/or 4+ servings of fruit per day.

B. sweeteners or foods made with sweeteners twice per day and/or 3+ servings of fruit per day.

C. sweeteners or foods made with sweeteners once per day and/or 2+ servings of fruit per day.

5. *My sugar and carb cravings are*

A. so strong that I'm admittedly fearful of how this detox will go for me.

B. pretty darned strong—that's why I'm reading this!

C. not terrible, but certainly apparent enough that I'm here!

If you answered mostly **A**, then select **Level 1**.

If you answered mostly **B**, then select **Level 2**.

If you answered mostly **C**, then select **Level 3**.

If, upon reviewing your resulting level, it seems more difficult than you are prepared for, you may default to the lower level. So, for example, if your test revealed you would be on Level 2 of the program but, upon reading the Yes/No Foods List, you think it'll simply be too difficult, you may complete Level 1. You are also welcome to include some of the allowed foods for your level on some days and not others. So, for example, if you are completing Level 1 or 2 and you simply don't eat dairy one day, that's completely fine. Once you complete the program at Level 2 successfully, you are welcome to follow Level 3 next time, should you decide to complete the program again in the future.

THE 21-DAY SUGAR DETOX Official Program Rules

YES TO ALL

LEVEL 1	LEVEL 2	LEVEL 3
Eggs Meat Seafood	Eggs Meat Seafood	Eggs Meat Seafood
Vegetables (Non-starchy & starchy, including potatoes and plantains)	Vegetables (Non-starchy & starchy, including potatoes and plantains)	Vegetables (Non-starchy & starchy, including potatoes and plantains)
Lemons and limes Nuts and seeds	Lemons and limes Nuts and seeds	Lemons and limes Nuts and seeds
Healthy fats, like those in meat, egg yolks, coconut oil, avocados, olive oil, and butter/ghee	Healthy fats, like those in meat, egg yolks, coconut oil, avocados, olive oil, and butter/ghee	Healthy fats, like those in meat, egg yolks, coconut oil, avocados, olive oil, and butter/ghee
Nut/coconut-based "dairy"	Nut/coconut-based "dairy"	Nut/coconut-based "dairy"
Coffee Tea Still & sparkling waters (unsweetened only) Vinegars Spices & herbs	Coffee Tea Still & sparkling waters (unsweetened only) Vinegars Spices & herbs	Coffee Tea Still & sparkling waters (unsweetened only) Vinegars Spices & herbs
Dairy, full-fat	Dairy, full-fat	

THE FOLLOWING FOODS HAVE PORTION LIMITS EACH DAY

LEVEL 1	LEVEL 2	LEVEL 3
Fruit *(1 piece per day total)* Choice of green apple, green-tipped/underripe banana, or grapefruit	Fruit *(1 piece per day total)* Choice of green apple, green-tipped/underripe banana, or grapefruit	Fruit *(1 piece per day total)* Choice of green apple, green-tipped/underripe banana, or grapefruit
Coconut water Kombucha *(8 ounces/day max each)*	Coconut water Kombucha *(8 ounces/day max each)*	Coconut water Kombucha *(8 ounces/day max each)*
Starch flours *(2 tablespoons/day max total)* Cassava, tapioca, arrowroot, etc.	Starch flours *(2 tablespoons/day max total)* Cassava, tapioca, arrowroot, etc.	Starch flours *(2 tablespoons/day max total)* Cassava, tapioca, arrowroot, etc.
Gluten-free grains or legumes *(½ cup per day max total)* Rice, quinoa, black beans, garbanzo beans, etc.		

NO TO ALL

LEVEL 1	LEVEL 2	LEVEL 3
Alcohol	Alcohol	Alcohol
Dairy, nonfat & low-fat	Dairy, nonfat & low-fat	Dairy, all
Fruits & fruit juices unless listed above	Fruits & fruit juices unless listed above	Fruits & fruit juices unless listed above
Gluten-containing grains	Gluten-containing grains	Gluten-containing grains
Gluten-free grain flours or flour-based foods	Gluten-free grains	Gluten-free grains
Soy	Soy	Soy
Sweeteners	Sweeteners	Sweeteners
Vegetable oils*	Vegetable oils*	Vegetable oils*

* These oils are nearly impossible to avoid when dining out, so the rules here are that they aren't allowed for use in your home or in prepackaged foods that are otherwise 21DSD-friendly. Refer to the Guide to Dining Out on page 108 for more tips on ordering 21DSD-friendly meals when you are away from home.

YES FOODS LEVELS 1, 2, & 3

Eat plenty of these foods for 21 days for all levels and without portion limits except where noted.

MEAT, FISH & EGGS

All meats, including deli meats and cured meats like bacon (OK if there's sugar in the cure), pancetta, and prosciutto

All fish & seafood

All eggs

NUTS/SEEDS
whole, flour, or butters

All nuts and seeds are included in all forms.

FRUIT

Lemons (unlimited)

Limes (unlimited)

Up to 1 piece per day of the below fruit is allowed, in any combination. For example, you may have ½ of a green-tipped banana and ½ of a green apple in one day.

Bananas, green-tipped / not quite ripe only

Grapefruit, any

Green / Granny Smith apples only

STARCHY VEGETABLES

Acorn squash

Beets

Butternut squash

Cassava *(or up to 2 tbsp max total starch flours per day)*

Green peas

Plantains

Pumpkin

Sweet potatoes, yams

Tapioca *(or up to 2 tbsp max total starch flours per day)*

Taro

White potatoes

Winter squash (assorted)

VEGETABLES

Artichokes/sunchokes

Asparagus

Broccoli

Brussels sprouts

Cabbage

Carrots

Cauliflower

Celery/celery root

Chard

Collards

Cucumber

Eggplant

Fennel

Garlic

Ginger

Green beans

Horseradish

Jicama

Kale

Leeks

Lettuce, all leafy greens

Mushrooms

Onions

Parsnips

Peppers, all varieties

Radicchio

Radishes

Rutabaga

Snow/snap peas

Spaghetti squash

Spinach

Tomato

Turnips

Yellow squash

Zucchini

FATS & OILS
see page 111

Animal fats such as duck fat, lard, schmaltz & tallow

Avocados, avocado oil

Coconut oil

Flax oil

Ghee, clarified butter

Olives, olive oil

Sesame oil

CONDIMENTS/MISC.

Broth (pp 244–245)

Coconut aminos

21DSD Ketchup (p 232) (no store-bought ketchups are allowed)

All flavor extracts

Mayonnaise made with olive or avocado oil or homemade (p 246); do your best to avoid others

Mustard, gluten-free varieties

Nutritional yeast

SALAD DRESSINGS

Read labels carefully; homemade is best (see pp 238–240)

SPICES & HERBS

All are OK; check premixed blends for hidden sugars

VINEGARS

Apple cider, balsamic, distilled, red wine, sherry, white

SUPPLEMENTS

Protein powder, 100% pure with NO other ingredients (e.g., 100% whey, collagen, gelatin, egg white, pea, or hemp)

Pure vitamin or mineral supplements

BEVERAGES— NOT SWEET

Almond milk, unsweetened or homemade (p 242)

Coconut milk, unsweetened, store-bought or homemade p 243)

Coconut cream, full-fat

Coffee, espresso

Mineral water

Seltzer, club soda

Teas: all unsweetened teas are okay

Water

BEVERAGES— NATURALLY SWEET

Up to 1 cup total per day is allowed, in any combination. For example, you may have ½ cup of coconut water and ½ cup of kombucha in one day.

Coconut juice, coconut water (no added sweeteners)

Kombucha, homebrewed or store-bought

PLUS, FOR **LEVEL 1** ONLY

GLUTEN-FREE GRAINS/LEGUMES

Up to ½ cup serving per day (cooked) is allowed of whole forms only—NO GRAIN- OR LEGUME-BASED FLOURS

Amaranth	Lentils
Arrowroot	Millet
Beans: black, fava, garbanzo (chickpeas) (up to ½ cup of hummus is okay), navy, pinto, red	Oats (steel-cut only)
	Quinoa
	Rice (brown, white, wild)
	Sorghum
Buckwheat	

FOR **LEVELS 1 & 2** ONLY

DAIRY

Full-fat (4% or higher) only!

Butter

Cheese, cream cheese, cottage cheese

Half & half

Heavy cream

Milk, whole only

Sour cream

Yogurt/kefir, plain

Refer to the short Finding Your Level quiz on page 18.

NO FOODS   Do not eat these foods for 21 days for all levels.

DAIRY

Level 1 & 2: all nonfat & low-fat dairy

Level 3: all dairy except butter/ghee

FOODS CONTAINING REFINED GRAINS

Bagels

Bread/breadsticks

Brownies

Cake

Candy

Cereal/granola

Chips

Cookies

Crackers

Croissants

Cupcakes

Muffins

Pasta

Pastries

Pita

Pizza

Popcorn

Rice cakes

Rolls

VEGETABLES/ STARCHES

Corn (whole, flour, polenta, grits, etc.)

Soybeans/edamame

FRUIT (fresh, dried, or other)

No fruit except what is on the Yes foods list

GRAINS/LEGUMES

Barley

Flours made from grains or beans (chickpeas, lentils, etc.)

Kamut

Oats (steel-cut oats are a Yes food for Level 1)

Pasta (all kinds, including couscous & orzo)

Rye

Soybeans/edamame (including miso, natto, soy sauce, tempeh, and tofu)

Spelt

Wheat

(No grains/legumes at all for Level 2 & 3.)

BEVERAGES

All alcohol

Coffee drinks or shakes, pre-sweetened

Juice

Milk: skim, nonfat, 1%, 2%, soy/rice/oat

Soda (regular & diet)

Sweet-tasting drinks (besides herbal teas)

CONDIMENTS/MISC.

Ketchup, store-bought

Mayonnaise, spreads, or salad dressings made with canola, soybean, or "vegetable" oil

Soy sauce, tamari

ANYTHING "DIET," SUGAR-FREE, OR ARTIFICIALLY SWEETENED

This means no chewing gum, either!

SWEETENERS OF ANY KIND

None are allowed!

SUPPLEMENTS

Anything that includes sugar, sweeteners, or sugar alcohols (xylitol, for example)

Protein powders that have more than one ingredient (see "supplements" on p 20)

Shakeology and similar blends

Supplements that contain soy, corn, or wheat

VEGETABLE OILS*

Man made buttery spreads, trans fats, hydrogenated or partially hydrogenated oils, margarine, "buttery spreads"

Canola oil

Corn oil

Grapeseed oil

Rice bran oil

Safflower oil

Soybean oil

Sunflower oil

*See "Guide to Healthy Fats & Oils" on p. 111.

Building Your 21DSD Plate

If you're struggling to feel satiated or your energy is low, you may need to rethink how much you're eating. Below are some examples of how to build your plate for the next three weeks.

EXAMPLE MEALS **LEVEL 1**

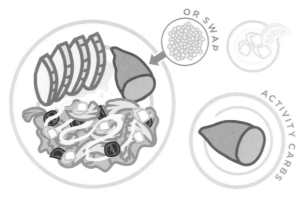

~4 ounces **protein**

1-2 cups **non-starchy vegetables**

1-2 tablespoons **healthy fats^**

optional ½-1 ounce **dairy**

optional ½ cup **starchy vegetables or whole gluten-free grains/legumes***

+ ACTIVITY CARBS *(see page 24)*
½-1 cup **starchy vegetables** in addition to the above per meal as needed

EXAMPLE MEALS **LEVEL 2**

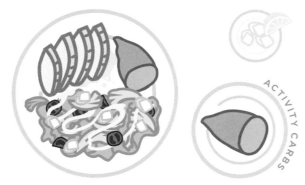

~4 ounces **protein**

1-2 cups **non-starchy vegetables**

1-2 tablespoons **healthy fats^**

optional ½-1 ounce **dairy**

optional ½ cup **starchy vegetables**

+ ACTIVITY CARBS *(see page 24)*
½-1 cup **starchy vegetables** in addition to the above per meal as needed

EXAMPLE MEALS **LEVEL 3**

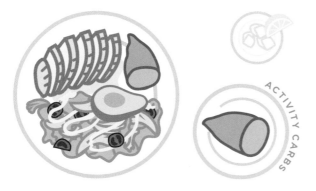

4-6 ounces **protein**

1-2 cups **non-starchy vegetables**

1-2 tablespoons **healthy fats^**

optional ½ cup **starchy vegetables**

+ ACTIVITY CARBS *(see page 24)*
½-1 cup **starchy vegetables** in addition to the above per meal as needed

---

^ See the Guide to Healthy Fats & Oils on page 111. Equivalent amounts of avocado (¼ or ½ avocado) or nuts/seeds (2 tablespoons) may also be used.

Please note that these are absolutely not prescriptive or intended to limit your portions (aside from foods that are only allowed in limited portions—see page 19). If you are able to easily build a plate with the foods included on the program and you feel good, these guidelines don't need to apply to you.

EXAMPLE SNACKS **LEVEL 1**

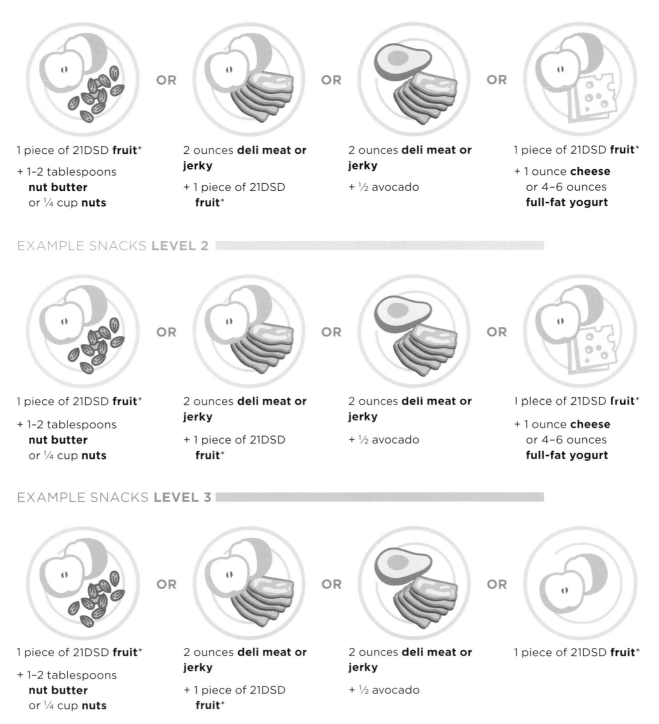

1 piece of 21DSD **fruit***

+ 1–2 tablespoons
   nut butter
   or ¼ cup **nuts**

OR

2 ounces **deli meat or jerky**

+ 1 piece of 21DSD
   fruit*

OR

2 ounces **deli meat or jerky**

+ ½ avocado

OR

1 piece of 21DSD **fruit***

+ 1 ounce **cheese**
   or 4–6 ounces
   full-fat yogurt

EXAMPLE SNACKS **LEVEL 2**

1 piece of 21DSD **fruit***

+ 1–2 tablespoons
   nut butter
   or ¼ cup **nuts**

OR

2 ounces **deli meat or jerky**

+ 1 piece of 21DSD
   fruit*

OR

2 ounces **deli meat or jerky**

+ ½ avocado

OR

1 piece of 21DSD **fruit***

+ 1 ounce **cheese**
   or 4–6 ounces
   full-fat yogurt

EXAMPLE SNACKS **LEVEL 3**

1 piece of 21DSD **fruit***

+ 1–2 tablespoons
   nut butter
   or ¼ cup **nuts**

OR

2 ounces **deli meat or jerky**

+ 1 piece of 21DSD
   fruit*

OR

2 ounces **deli meat or jerky**

+ ½ avocado

OR

1 piece of 21DSD **fruit***

---

* Follow daily portion limits. Your daily portions may be eaten in one sitting or divided among your meals and snack.

FAQs

Q: *How many meals should I eat each day?*

A: I recommend that most people eat three full meals per day plus one snack. If that doesn't work for your lifestyle or appetite, you can choose to eat two larger meals and two snacks, or two larger meals and one snack, or no snacks. Just be sure that you are not undereating, which can make you feel tired, hungry, or weak.

Q: *Do I need to eat the included snacks? Can I have more than one snack per day?*

A: No, you do not *need* to eat snacks. You can enjoy your daily piece of fruit as part of a meal or recipe (e.g., in a smoothie, chopped up and put into a salad, or on yogurt for breakfast). You may also find that your meals are extremely satiating and you don't need a snack. Eat a small portion of food (a snack) if you are hungry between meals, but don't eat it simply because it's there. Snacks are listed simply as guidelines and recommendations for what to eat if you feel you need them—they are not required. And if you're hungry, you can have more than one snack, as long as you don't have more than one piece of fruit each day.

Q: *Am I required to eat my included fruit for the day? Can I eat half a piece of one type of fruit and half a piece of another?*

A: No, you don't have to eat your allotted piece of fruit each day. However, you cannot carry over uneaten fruit to the following day. There's no rollover fruit! So if you choose not to eat your green apple today, for example, you can't add it to tomorrow's meals. You may have one piece total per day, or leave it out—that's up to you. You may split your fruit portions between half a piece of one kind and half a piece of another within one day if you choose. So, for example, you may eat half of a green apple and half of a green-tipped banana in one day.

Q: (Level 1) *Am I required to eat ½ cup of gluten-free grains or legumes for the day? Can I eat ¼ cup of one type and ¼ cup of another?*

A: No, you don't have to eat your daily ½ cup of gluten-free grains or legumes. However, you cannot carry over what you don't eat to the following day. You're welcome to eat a combination of different gluten-free grains or legumes, as long as the total amount you eat doesn't exceed ½ cup per day.

Q: *What are activity carbs, and who should add them?*

A: Activity carbs are starchy vegetables that people who meet certain criteria should eat in addition to standard 21DSD plate portions. Anyone who exercises or is active throughout the day, naturally very lean people (ectomorphs or "hardgainers"), pregnant and breastfeeding moms, and anyone who generally *feels better* eating more healthy carbs must add activity carbs. There is no reason to avoid these carbs if you feel better eating them. Your 21DSD will *not* be derailed by adding them (a common misconception). In fact, you will be more successful if you add these healthy carbs because you'll feel a lot better, and eating healthy carbs when your body needs them keeps more cravings at bay!

Q: *Why are some items listed as optional?*

A: Just because a food or food group is permitted doesn't mean that you *must* include it every day or in every meal. While you are permitted to include up to ½ cup per day of gluten-free grains or legumes on Level 1, for example, there is no requirement for you to eat them. You can opt for starchy vegetables instead on some days, or most days, or not. On Levels 1 and 2, dairy is another optionally added food—meaning you can include it in some meals or not. Whether or not you eat the optional items won't affect the success of your 21DSD.

Q: *What is a non-starchy vegetable?*

A: Anything leafy, green, and relatively low in carbohydrates per serving is considered a non-starchy vegetable. So, for example, lettuce, spinach, kale, Brussels sprouts, cabbage, green beans, cauliflower, bell peppers, onions, jicama, and carrots (yes, even carrots) are all non-starchy vegetables.

Q: *What is a starchy vegetable?*

A: Anything that is higher in carbohydrates and has a starchy texture is a starchy vegetable. So, for example, sweet potatoes, potatoes, yams, butternut/winter squash, beets, and plantains are all starchy vegetables.

Q: *Why does Level 3 have larger protein portions?*

A: Since Level 3 is dairy-free and dairy is a source of protein (and fat) for those in Levels 1 and 2, those following Level 3 may find that increasing their protein intake from meat or eggs is more satiating.

Q: *What if I can't eat certain 21DSD-friendly foods or I'm allergic to the included fruits? Can I swap some foods out for others?*

A: If you are allergic to certain foods that are specified on the plan, such as green apples, then omit those foods and simply eat from the list of Yes foods. You may not switch the included fruits out for others. Don't worry, you can enjoy a perfectly successful detox without those foods. There is no reason why you must have fruit, or any specific foods, while on the program.

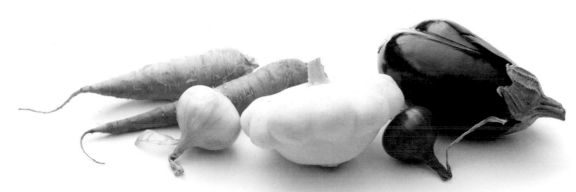

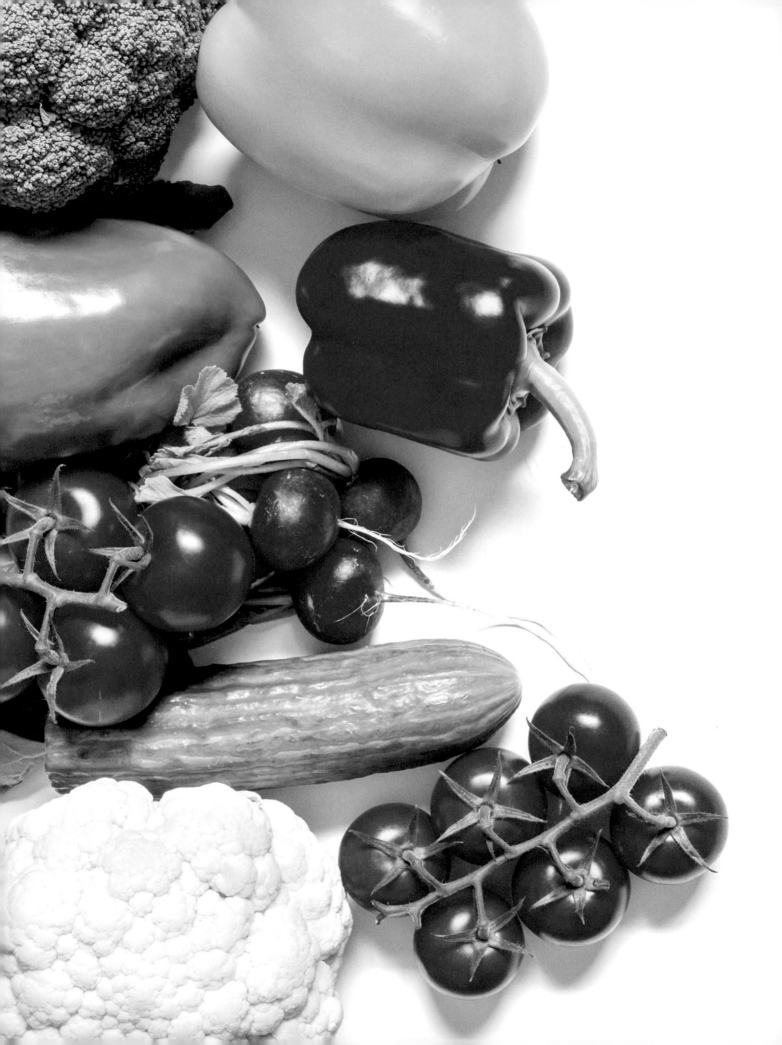

MINDSET:
A ROAD MAP FOR SUCCESS

In hundreds of thousands of 21DSD participants, I've seen two main factors to success on the program:

1) **The practical side:** Your actions; preparation and follow-through—shopping for and prepping your food, previewing restaurant menus, preparing for travel or social gatherings, and so on.

2) **The mental side:** Your thoughts; maintaining positive self-talk, listening to the "I can do this!" part of you that knows, for sure, that you *can* do hard things—and that, with the help of this book, it'll be much, much easier.

If the practical side seems overwhelming, take heart, because the day-by-day guide in this book covers *everything* you need to do. It tells you not just what recipes are planned for each day but also how to cook extra and use leftovers to remix into a new dish, what to cook in advance to make meal prep easier, what to buy for the week ahead, and more—you are totally covered!

If the mental side is throwing you for a loop—you're worried about whether you can commit to and follow through with this, even though you've decided you *want* to—I hear you! It's completely normal to be thinking about the reasons why you haven't committed to this program until now. But there are things you can do to change your mindset and prepare yourself for success. In this section, I'll explain the most common mental roadblocks and how to handle them.

I promise you this: you are *fully capable* of doing this program.

I want to approach this in the most positive way I can, but it's important to acknowledge what some of the most common fears are, so that you know you're not alone here. Know that when I list something as a "mindset roadblock," it's entirely something you control based upon your beliefs. Unlike practical blocks to your success, which can be overcome with hands-on, action-based tasks, these roadblocks require you to change your thinking.

THE 3 MINDSET ROADBLOCKS

1. LACK OF SUPPORT

I don't think I can do this on my own.

I don't have the support I need.

I need a lot of support!

2. OTHER PEOPLE'S THOUGHTS AND FEELINGS

I'm worried about what people will say or think.

How will I answer when my coworker asks me why I'm not drinking alcohol at happy hour?

It's easier to eat the cake than to explain why I'm not eating it.

3. FEAR OF FAILURE

What if I'm not perfect?

What if I slip up or lack the discipline and willpower it takes to do this?

What if I fail?

I'm going to dig into each of these three mindset roadblocks, reframe them, and give you some strategies for tackling them.

Lack of support

Certainly, having a supportive spouse, partner, roommate, and/or family makes this program a whole lot easier. But we're each in control of our own lives. Yes, we live with other people. Yes, we are influenced by other people. And, yes, our choices can be made easier with the support of those around us. However, there are likely actions you take every single day that your loved ones don't also take. There are activities you enjoy that they don't. There are television shows you enjoy that they don't. There are foods you currently eat and love that they don't.

REALITY CHECK

You are in control of your own thoughts and actions.

You are responsible for your own thoughts and actions.

When you wrap up your ability to succeed on the 21DSD in whether or not those immediately around you are on board, you're handing someone else more power over your life. You are autonomous! No, lack of support doesn't make your program easier, but you certainly don't need everyone to support you in order to be firm in your decision and convictions about what is best for you.

Furthermore, if you're in a situation where you're hoping to encourage those around you to eventually complete this program themselves, a consistently positive attitude in the absence of their support will only strengthen your case.

WHAT WILL MY SPOUSE/PARTNER/FAMILY EAT IF I'M EATING 21DSD MEALS THAT THEY DON'T LIKE?

Let me start by saying that the food on the 21DSD is seriously delicious, bold, and healthy. It isn't diet food. Many participants over the years have easily assimilated 21DSD recipes right into their daily routines without much problem at all. If you don't mention that a meal is "detox food," your family probably won't notice anything has changed. (And to answer a frequent question: yes, even very young children like these meals. Thousands of parents have fed them to their kids with great success.)

That said, I get it. It's likely that a lot of your usual meals relied heavily on refined carbs—like pizza, or takeout, or sandwiches, pastries, cereal … The list goes on.

It seems at first like there are two choices: you can cook two separate meals, or you can let your family know that you're making a 21DSD meal and they can take it or leave it. But there's also a middle ground that I think can work well to keep the peace: cook your 21DSD meal, but add in a little bit of non-21DSD foods along with them for others in your family.

For example, perhaps your family is not very excited about spaghetti squash or zoodles (though I'll always argue that it wouldn't hurt to try them a few times!). You can easily make 80 to 90 percent of the meal 21DSD-friendly, then simply add pasta noodles to their portions to keep them happy.

I'm not saying you should become a short-order cook and be at the beck and call of everyone around you. But it comes down to either finding a middle ground (which, yes, may involve cooking more) or holding your ground, cooking the meal you want to eat, and letting your family decide whether to eat it or not.

It's worth the effort to at least try to feed your family the healthiest food you can while making it taste great. What do you have to lose?

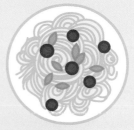

If you're thinking that you'll need lots of support to help you on the 21DSD, I first want to commend you on some really solid self-knowledge! Knowing what you need to be successful is one of the most critical pieces of information you can have.

So let's think about strategies for getting you the support you need:

1. Use what you've got! There is so, so, so much support available for this program if you look for it. If you're not getting support from family and friends around you, enlist a friend in another city who can do the program with you and text about it. Or find a coworker who has been talking about wanting to quit eating so much sugar.

2. Reach out to our community. Folks around the world are completing this challenge every month and sharing about it online. Look for the hashtag #21DSD on social media, join the 21-Day Sugar Detox Community group on Facebook, and follow the @21daysugardetox Instagram account. There's also an optional online program that complements this book, complete with a daily email series and a lot of helpful videos (visit 21dsd.com for details).

   Whether you find a social media–based buddy or a fellow member of the online program, there are countless people who can help and encourage you, even if they're not right in your own home.

3. Enlist the outside accountability of a Certified 21DSD Coach! Surf on over to 21dsd.com/coaches and you'll likely find a coach near you, or, if not super local to you, one who offers virtual coaching. Our Certified Coaches all go through a training program specifically for the 21DSD and have all completed the program themselves—plus, there are coaches who specialize in particular concerns, like athletic performance or autoimmunity. And if you can find a local event or group that will meet in person near you, don't hesitate to go—you'll have an amazing experience!

   Who knows, maybe you'll be so inspired by your experience with your coach, you'll become a coach yourself!

Mindset Roadblock #2:
Other People's Thoughts and Feelings

For some reason, many of us put a lot of our own self-worth in other people's hands. We base how we feel about ourselves on what they think of us.

Now, in some areas of life, weighing the thoughts and feelings of others is perfectly valid. But your own self-improvement is not one of those areas. When other people's thoughts and feelings (which I'm going to call "OPTF") get between you and your own goals, that's where we all need to draw the line.

Anytime someone is not in favor your growth, self-improvement, or pursuit of better health, I recommend seriously questioning whether or not their opinion is relevant or valid. Why do they get to have an opinion on something that is about you and your own life? Chances are, you'll realize that their opinion is not, in fact, relevant, helpful, or constructive. It's a bold statement, but sometimes even your parents, sweetheart, and closest friends simply shouldn't have a say, especially when their input is going to bring you down.

REALITY CHECK

Your decision not to eat or drink something is no one's business but your own.

If you don't make a big deal of your choices around the house or at an event, there's a much better chance that others will also see it as a non-issue.

What if people question what you're eating (or not eating)? You have my permission to dismiss OPTF when it comes to improving your own health! Of course, this doesn't mean that you get to be inconsiderate, rude, or offensive. It simply means that you do not need to answer to anyone other than yourself.

I know that it can be tough to handle what someone else may say about what you're choosing in the heat of the moment. Even if you're doing your best to keep to yourself or simply hold your ground, other people may challenge your choices. Here are some strategies for handling OPTF:

1. Remember that you only have control over yourself. You can't control or change someone else's thoughts. Often people feel as if your choice to eat something healthy means you are judging them for their own food choices— which must be something you believe is unhealthy, since you aren't eating it, and therefore you must believe *they* are bad or unhealthy as well. We both know that you aren't thinking that. We both know that what you're really thinking is, "Well, if I wasn't on this detox, I'd be throwing back the wine right there with you!" Simply hold your ground if you are confronted—which brings me to point 2.

2. Keep the focus on yourself. No matter what you do, some people will still question what you're doing and even criticize you. Your best defense is to stay focused on why you are simply "eating foods that feel best for you right now." No one can question or object to how much better you feel eating the way you choose to eat right now. Conversation over. Change the subject or walk away from it.

3. Be delicate about what you're doing. Be aware of the words you choose and make it a point *not* to say things about what anyone else is eating that may come across as judgmental. This can be difficult, but it's best to understand that not every "healthy" choice is right for everyone else. Some people can eat foods that cause cravings or uncontrollable eating patterns for you without experiencing these things. There's no need to assume that what you're doing is right for them, so tread lightly and stay focused on your own needs.

Mindset Roadblock #3:
Fear of failure

REALITY CHECK

When we say we're afraid to fail, what we really mean is this: we don't believe we can maintain the discipline and willpower necessary to achieve our goal.

If you think about it, at the root of a fear of failure isn't the actual "failing" itself, since that's a very intangible result, right? What does it even mean to fail on the 21DSD? Does it mean you didn't do it "properly" or didn't finish? Or that you "slipped up" or weren't perfect?

Sit with that for a moment.

At some point in your life, you achieved something you didn't think you could. You did something hard. And you did that through discipline and willpower—even if now you don't think it was as difficult to achieve as completing the 21DSD. So you've certainly shown that you have discipline and willpower in the past, and I believe you can have them again right now.

But, as you may imagine, discipline and willpower are not things you can simply decide to have; you have to make a consistent effort at strengthening them, much like muscles in your body. So the best way to combat concern over a lack of discipline or willpower is preparation! While this *is* a mindset roadblock, the way to overcome it is by doing the actions outlined in this guide every day.

If the discipline and willpower needed to follow the plan seem overwhelming, I have a handful of specific strategies for you:

1. Focus on the now. Instead of thinking about completing twenty-one days, take the program just three or four days at a time. Most of the shopping, prep work, and cooking are done for those three or four days. There's no need to overwhelm yourself by reading too far ahead or anticipating the challenges of days far in the future. Tackle each day as it comes and think about just the next few days ahead of you.

2. Define your "why" and revisit it as needed. To stay motivated, it's critical that the reason you are doing this program is meaningful to you. You cannot be completing this program for a reason that doesn't feel 100 percent real and true for you. Whether you want to heal your body of a health challenge like type 2 diabetes or prediabetes, for example, or you simply want to feel less controlled by sugar and carbs, your personal reason for completing this program needs to be powerful to you. Solidarity—completing the program alongside a close friend, coworker, or loved one—may be a strong enough "why" for you, but it may not! Be sure that your "why" feels compelling; otherwise, it isn't likely to stick.

3. Flip the script! If temptation for off-plan foods arises, try repeating these mantras: "This food is not special," or "I can have it later if I decide I want it, but not right now." No, really—we can all have pretty much any food we want, anytime we want (thanks, Internet!). Sure, we may have to go through some effort to make it or shop somewhere different to buy it, but it really isn't special. It can feel special because it's being served at an event, or at a restaurant, or by a special person, but the food itself is not special. And you really *can* have it later if you want it, but right now, you've made a commitment and you're sticking to it!

4. The best defense is a good offense. Remove temptation from your home or office desk (since you can't take all office treats away, obviously). I'll talk about this a lot in the daily guides, but remember that creating the environment that you need to support yourself is a huge element of building discipline.

   Don't arrive hungry at a party or social event and then act surprised if there's nothing 21DSD-friendly for you to eat. If you don't already know, I'll tell you right now: party food often does not align well with healthy, real food. I've got lots of practical tips for you on managing parties, choosing 21DSD-friendly foods, and more on page 108.

I won't tell you that the 21DSD isn't a challenge—it definitely is. But it's very achievable! If you recognize any of your own mindset roadblocks in the list above, take heart; many people with these exact same roadblocks have successfully completed the 21DSD. You can do it too: own your choices, be prepared, and stay strong!

THE
WEEK
BEFORE
YOUR
DETOX

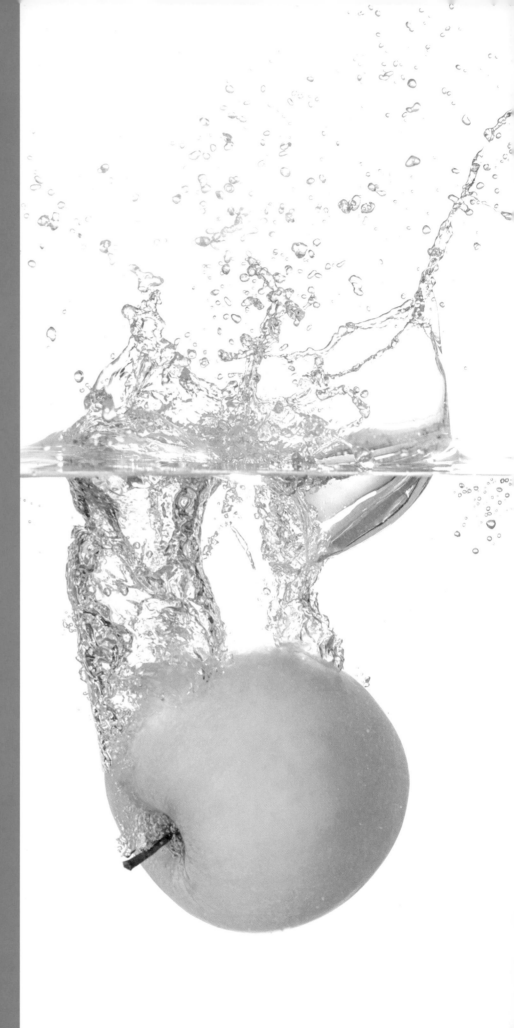

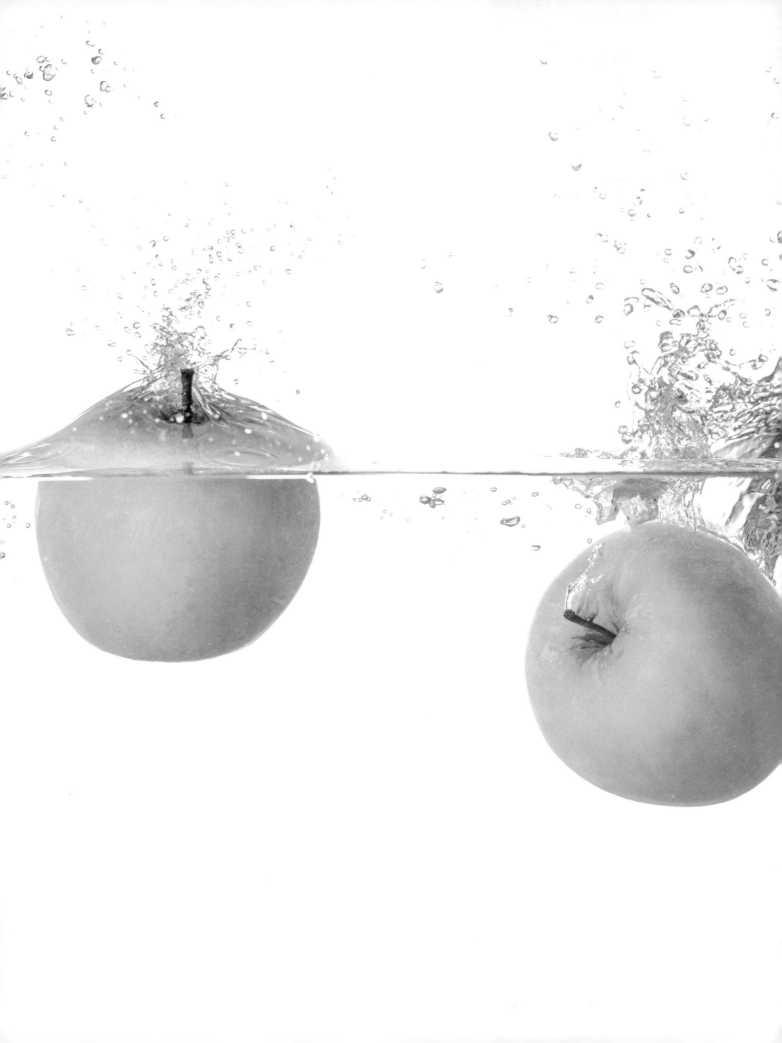

WHAT TO EXPECT

"I'm totally excited for this, I think . . . "

Feelings of anxiety and nervousness are typical when you decide to embark on the 21DSD program. Taking the coming week to prepare and learn about sugar will help you get ready for day 1. No need to worry, just stay with me each day!

The Dish from Diane

A week out from your 21DSD, you're filled with blind optimism. At this point, you are probably nervous about how you'll succeed. But at the same time you're feeling so ready for this change—in fact, you wonder if you really need an entire week of prep. All I can say is this: trust the process. As you head into this week, keep in mind that the efforts you make now will help you truly succeed over the twenty-one days. Inevitably, those who commit to the program one day and then start it the next . . . well, they fail. This program requires that you prepare for it, and when you're truly ready, your commitment will pay off!

TODAY'S CHECKLIST

- [ ] **Read the complete introduction** to this book (pages 5–15).

- [ ] **Review the Yes/No Foods List** (pages 19–21) and take note of No foods that you currently eat regularly.

- [ ] **Determine your level** (page 18) and take note of Yes/No foods that apply to you.

- [ ] **Build your 21DSD Plate** (pages 22–23) and anticipate how your meals and snacks will look. You can adjust these as necessary, but get a good starting point sorted out now.

- [ ] **Review the layout** of the daily pages and familiarize yourself with the meal plan format.

TODAY'S LESSON

Why do we crave sugar?

Long ago, the only sweet-tasting foods available were fruit and honey, which were nutrient-dense and available only seasonally. Therefore, our ancestors ate far fewer calories from sweet foods than we do today, when we have sugar-laced foods available to us all the time.

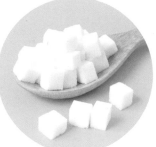

Why are we wired to love and seek out sweet foods? If we know sugar is bad for us, why do we constantly want to eat it?

The answer: DOPAMINE! Dopamine is a neurotransmitter that helps to control feelings of reward and pleasure. We get dopamine hits from many healthy sources, such as physical touch and exercise, but unfortunately, we also see a spike in dopamine when we have caffeine, narcotics, and—you guessed it—sugar.

When we eat sugar, the dopamine response we get encourages us to continually search for that pleasurable feeling. This wouldn't be an inherently bad thing if you were receiving these signals from eating nutrient-dense sources of sugar, like berries, in the context of an overall healthy, balanced diet.

But that's not what happens today. Today, it's most often refined forms of sugar that are empty of nutrients that are triggering the release of dopamine, which leaves you with a constant desire for more sugar!

WHAT I ATE TODAY

Right now, for your pre-detox week, simply write down what you are eating, but don't try to follow any of the detox rules yet! This is for your information and for reference after your detox, so you can look back and compare your food choices before and after.

B: _____   D: _____

_____   _____

L: _____   S: _____

_____   _____

6 DAYS Pre-Detox

TODAY'S LESSON
Where sugar hides

Even foods that are not considered "sweet" or "treats" can have sugar hiding in their ingredients! Sugar may be sneaking into your grocery cart through some unexpected (but very common) suspects.

Take these three examples:

1. Boxed cereals: Sugar is usually in these products—even those that are considered healthy—in at least two different forms, like honey or cane sugar and brown rice syrup.

2. Salad dressings: Most premade salad dressings have added sugar. Even worse, the diet varieties have artificial sweeteners. To make your own salad dressing, you just need oil, vinegar or lemon/lime juice, spices, and maybe some mustard—not sugar! Use the recipes on pages 238–240 for your salads while on the 21DSD.

3. Pasta sauces: Pasta sauce can be a perfectly healthy and delicious option when done right (as in the recipe on page 237), especially over zoodles (zucchini noodles) and spaghetti squash. (As you probably guessed, pasta made from refined flour is out on the 21DSD.) But most store-bought pasta sauces contain added sugar: to cover up some less-than-ripe tomatoes going into the sauce, to act as a preservative, or even as a flavor enhancer. Any way you cut it, it's totally unnecessary.

Here's a super-sneaky sugar secret: food manufacturers often use multiple types of sweeteners to avoid listing a single sweetener as the first (that is, the most abundant) item in the ingredient list. In other words, if they were to use just one sweetener, it would be the first ingredient because there's more sweetener than any other ingredient. Using multiple sweeteners means there's less of each, so they're further down the list. Most people know to check the first couple ingredients, so by putting several sweeteners way down in the list, food manufacturers can make the food look healthier than it is. This is also a sneaky way to use less of an expensive sweetener, like honey, and still be able to claim the food is "sweetened with honey," which sounds much better than "sweetened with high-fructose corn syrup."

There are also more than fifty ways to list sweeteners in an ingredients list without the word "sugar" ever appearing. It can show up as syrups, malts, molasses, sorbitol, juices, and way more. Use the Guide to Hidden Sugars on page 109 as your reference until you learn the most common offenders hiding in ingredient lists.

WHAT I ATE TODAY

B: _____

_____

L: _____

D: _____

_____

S: _____

WHAT TO EXPECT

"Geez, sugar is in everything!"

You may feel frustrated and annoyed when you go through your pantry and see how many food manufacturers add sugar (in its many forms) to their products. Use this moment to appreciate how much you are already learning from the program!

The Dish from Diane

It's important to spend this week "building your why"—exploring the foundational information you need to make your commitment (why the program takes twenty-one days, why it's a "detox," why sugar is harmful, and so on) as well as thinking about your *personal* why. Starting this program with a strong sense of why you're doing it will help you stay motivated and inspired throughout the program. Is it to crush your cravings? To free yourself from the sweets and treats that call you into the pantry or fridge every day? Is it to gain energy? Improve your sleep? Feel better in your own skin? Support and inspire a friend who is also completing the program? Set a good example for your family/kids? *What is your why?* We'll talk more about this the day before you start the detox (page 40), but spend this week thinking about it so you'll already have some ideas when it comes time to fully articulate your why.

TODAY'S CHECKLIST

☐ **Pantry cleanout day!** Using the Yes/No Foods List (pages 19–21) and information on hidden sugars from today's lesson, check your pantry and fridge for off-plan ingredients and foods. Set them aside in your fridge or pantry and plan to remove them the day before you start the 21DSD. If you don't want to throw them away, you can donate them or set them somewhere safely out of reach for the duration of the 21DSD.

☐ **Read and review the Guide to Hidden Sugars** on page 109.

☐ **Follow @21daysugardetox and @dianesanfilippo on social media!** (See page 15 for all the 21DSD account links.)

WHAT TO EXPECT

"Do I really need to get rid of everything tempting?"

You may feel like it's unnecessary to get rid of the cookies or crackers in the pantry or the ice cream in your freezer, but when you arrive home after a long, stressful day at work on day 5 of your 21DSD, you're going to be happy they aren't sitting there to tempt you.

The Dish from Diane

Now is the time to take stock of what you eat regularly. It's likely going to change a lot over the course of this detox. Swapping out old pantry or fridge staples for healthier, 21DSD-friendly versions will set you up for success. Rather than feeling like there's nothing left to eat, you'll have lots of new, exciting things to try. Who doesn't like fun new foods?!

TODAY'S CHECKLIST

☐ **Review the Guide to Simple Swaps (page 110).** Identify simple 21DSD-friendly swaps for No foods you currently eat. Circle pantry items you'll need for the swaps on the shopping list.

☐ **Order pantry items online (if necessary).** If you are following the meal plan and can't find all of the pantry items locally, now's the time to order items on the shopping list from an online vendor. Even if you aren't following the meal plan, pantry staples are great to order ahead of time so you're not stuck without them mid-detox!

☐ **Order supplements you plan to use while on the program.** *These are totally optional* and not required at all to successfully complete the 21DSD, but many participants have said they help a ton. If you think you'll want the extra support, get on it now! (See pages 106–107 for the 21DSD guide to supplements.)

5 DAYS Pre-Detox

TODAY'S LESSON
Modify your meals

Don't miss out on foods you love! Yes, some of your usual favorites won't be included on the 21DSD, but I've got you covered! Rather than feeling down about not having cereal at breakfast or pasta at dinner, check out the swaps you can make that'll keep you full and satisfied. For example, instead of a grain-based granola, I'm serving up a healthy-fats punch with a nut-based granola (page 147). No spaghetti? No problem! You've got options like spaghetti squash or zoodles (page 174)—or even carrot noodles. Whatever you enjoy eating now that isn't included on the program, there's a healthy, 21DSD-friendly swap for it! Check out the guide on page 110 for more 21DSD swap ideas.

Swapping out these foods lets you find similar but healthier foods you love that can take their place. In order to carry the healthy habits you learn on the program into your everyday life, you need to truly enjoy what you're eating. And if your food on the 21DSD looks completely different from what you eat when you're not on the program, it's going to feel that much harder. The closer you can bring your 21DSD foods to something that looks (and tastes!) like foods you enjoy eating regularly, the easier it will be for you to stick with eating these foods in the long term.

KITCHEN TIP

Food storage containers make life so much easier on the 21DSD. If you don't already have a good supply, I recommend grabbing some larger, meal-sized containers, as well as smaller ones for things like sauces, chopped nuts, and on-the-go snacks. Zip-top bags in various sizes can also be really helpful, including both the large 1-gallon size, for things like prewashed and prepped greens, and the super-small 1-cup size, which can hold your jerky or other healthy snacks.

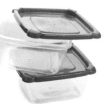

WHAT I ATE TODAY

B: _____

_____

L: _____

D: _____

_____

S: _____

4 DAYS Pre-Detox

TODAY'S LESSON
Artificial sweeteners

On page 35, we talked about forms of sugar you'll find on ingredient labels, like syrups, molasses, malts, and more. But we also need to address artificial sweeteners. These include acesulfame potassium (also known as acesulfame K, Sweet One, Sunett), aspartame (Equal, NutraSweet), saccharine (Sweet'N Low), and sucralose (Splenda). Note that while green stevia is a natural sweetener, when a stevia-containing product is white or presented in blended forms (Truvia), it may present problems similar to those of artificial sweeteners and should be consumed with caution if introduced or reintroduced (post detox).

Artificial sweeteners may cause health problems, including but not limited to:

- migraines and headaches
- dizziness and poor equilibrium
- convulsions and seizures
- nausea and vomiting
- diarrhea
- fatigue and weakness
- changes in mood
- changes in vision
- changes in heart rate
- joint pain
- memory loss
- sleep problems and insomnia
- hives and rashes
- weight-loss resistance

If you are suffering from any of these symptoms, I recommend kicking artificial sweeteners to the curb. And, since they're out for your 21DSD, now's the perfect time to quit them for good!

WHAT I ATE TODAY

B: _____

_____

L: _____

_____

D: _____

_____

S: _____

_____

WHAT TO EXPECT

"I'm savoring these last couple days of [insert favorite non-detox food]!"

As you start thinking about how your meals will change, you may find that you are enjoying your non-detox-approved foods. But by day 21, you won't even miss them! Don't worry, we'll talk about how and when (and maybe why not) to reintroduce your favorites after the detox ends, to see how you feel eating them.

The Dish from Diane

Remember when you dive into this detox that you are *choosing* this! When you interact with those around you who may not be supportive of it (because there's bound to be someone!), keep a positive attitude. If you complain the entire time you're on this program, what message does that send to your friends and loved ones you were probably trying to encourage to do this program with you? You got it: not a good one. What's more? When we tell ourselves a negative story, it becomes more and more true—so keep a positive mental outlook and your detox will go much more smoothly!

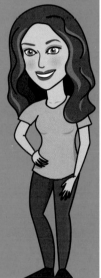

TODAY'S CHECKLIST

☐ **Perform a final sweep of your fridge** and pantry and double-check for artificial sweeteners or other ingredients that are going to be off-plan.

☐ **Log your food at left** and, using yesterday's lesson and the Guide to Simple Swaps (page 110), begin thinking of 21DSD-approved food swaps that you might enjoy in place of some of what you ate.

"Let the prepping begin!"

Now that you are just a few days out, it's a good idea to start prepping some of the recipe basics you'll be using the first week, such as ketchup (page 232). This will help keep you from feeling overwhelmed as day 1 approaches.

The Dish from Diane

As you move through this program, remember that carbs are not the enemy! While I talk a lot about how you may feel as a result of overdoing it with "bad carbs"—processed, refined foods without many nutrients—relative to your activity level and individual metabolism, this program isn't a war on carbs. Eating real, whole, nutrient-dense forms of carbohydrates, like sweet potatoes, isn't what has made us fatter and sicker over the years. And it certainly isn't what drives us to crave sugar and carbs every day! "Good carbs" like these have their place and aren't to be feared or avoided. Don't forget to use the guide to building your 21DSD plate on pages 22 to 23 to determine your starting plate and how to adjust it based on how you feel day-to-day.

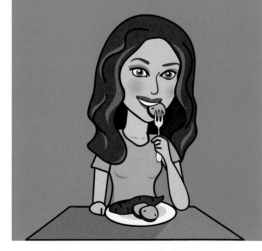

TODAY'S CHECKLIST

☐ **Log your food at right** and, using the Guide to Simple Swaps (page 110), begin thinking of 21DSD-approved food swaps that you might enjoy in place of some of what you ate.

3 DAYS Pre-Detox

TODAY'S LESSON
Carbs and your body, part 1

Carbohydrate is a macronutrient, along with protein and fat. Anything you eat that is not a protein or fat is a carbohydrate—from bread, pasta, rice, and candy to broccoli, butternut squash, berries, and basil. (Yes, there's a bit of protein and fat in those foods, but their major macronutrient is carbohydrate.)

When you eat carbohydrates, your body breaks them down into a usable form of energy called glucose. You can't keep more than four grams of glucose in your bloodstream at any given time; it needs to be either used or stored. That's where insulin comes in. Insulin is a hormone released by your pancreas when you eat carbohydrates. Its job is to tell your cells to let nutrients (including glucose) in.

Your brain and your red blood cells get first dibs on glucose, so before anything else happens, your liver, which is the master regulator of blood glucose levels, runs a check to make sure that your brain and red blood cells get what they need. Then your body can move on to using or storing the remaining glucose, moving it from your bloodstream into your body's "storage bins": your liver and your muscles. Glucose that is put into those storage bins is called glycogen.

As you eat more and more carbohydrates, your body responds with more and more insulin to help store that glucose for later use. There's a catch, though: your liver and muscles have limited storage space for carbohydrates (the exact amount varies from person to person). What happens to the carbohydrates that don't fit? They become…fat.

Stay tuned tomorrow for part 2 of carbs and your body!

WHAT I ATE TODAY

B: _____

_____

L: _____

D: _____

_____

S: _____

2 DAYS Pre-Detox

TODAY'S LESSON
Carbs and your body, part 2

I ended yesterday's lesson by talking about what happens when you consume more carbohydrates than your body can use for activity/exercise or store in the liver and muscles as glycogen: it's converted to fat! While the body has limited storage for carbohydrates, it has unlimited storage for fat—sneaky, right? This fat is in the form of either (1) triglycerides, which are fats that circulate in the blood, or (2) adipose, which is body fat.

Your total carbohydrate storage capacity = liver storage + muscle storage + carbohydrates you burn in a day (that's your resting metabolic rate plus any carbs you burn with activity or exercise).

If the amount of carbohydrates eaten is greater than liver storage + muscle storage + carbohydrates you burn in a day, then your body has no choice but to store the excess as fat. How and where you store your extra fat is determined largely by genetic predisposition.

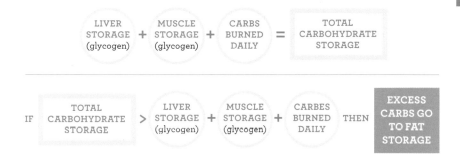

So how do you make sure that your body isn't getting more carbohydrates than it needs and converting all the excess to fat? It's a matter of the kinds of carbs you eat—processed and refined ("bad") or whole and nutrient-dense ("good")—as well as your activity level. Your body's system works smoothly and efficiently when the carbohydrates you eat are appropriate for your daily energy needs *and* come packaged as nature intended, with the vitamins and minerals required for the metabolism of carbohydrates. The 21-Day Sugar Detox includes only these good carbs, along with quality protein and fat.

WHAT I ATE TODAY

B: _____

L: _____

D: _____

S: _____

WHAT TO EXPECT

"I'm starting to get anxious. Can I really make it through this detox?!"

It's getting closer, so anxiety is natural, especially if this is your first 21DSD. But look at all of the prep work you have already completed and everything you have learned this week. You are ready for this new journey.

The Dish from Diane

Just. Breathe. You've got one more day to prepare before the detox begins. If you're planning to follow the meal plan (page 115), make sure to prepare the foods I'm outlining for you before day 1! I promise that you'll feel so much calmer and ready if you've got a fridge full of delicious food ready to go. The number one reason why people fail on any new nutritional program is failure to prepare—don't let it happen to you!

> "The greatest discovery of all time is that a person can change his future by merely changing his attitude."
>
> —Oprah Winfrey

TODAY'S CHECKLIST

- [ ] **Review Building Your 21DSD Plate** (pages 22–23) to be sure you're planning enough good carbs for your activity level.

- [ ] **Log your food** and rebuild your meals using 21DSD-approved food swaps.

- [ ] **Prep** ingredients for cooking tomorrow following the meal plan on page 115.

WHAT TO EXPECT

"Is my fridge going to be this full for the next three weeks?!"

You are probably feeling excited, anxious...and even busy! Approach the 21DSD feeling hopeful and positive. A good attitude is the best foundation, along with all of the planning and prep you have done. Now, time to clean up the kitchen!

The Dish from Diane

This book walks you through exactly what you need to do—and when—to succeed on the 21DSD. But no one can do it for you! You've got to stick to each day's plan and prep list, read the materials I present to you, and find answers to your questions right here as you go to keep your 21DSD running smoothly. This program is *yours*, and no one can be responsible for your success other than you. It's up to you to make it happen!

TODAY'S CHECKLIST

- [ ] **Log your food** and rebuild your meals using 21DSD-approved food swaps (see the Guide to Simple Swaps on page 110).

- [ ] **Prep** meals and meal components according to the meal plan on page 115.

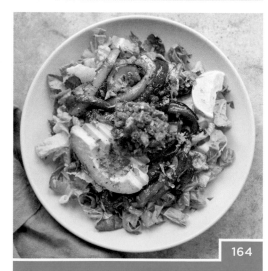

164

TODAY'S RECIPE
Chicken Fajita Salad

1 DAY Pre-Detox

TODAY'S LESSON
Setting goals and determining your why

Clearly, the central goal for completing the 21-Day Sugar Detox is to get sugar and bad carbs out of your life for the three weeks of the program. And, most likely, you also have a goal of reevaluating your dietary habits after the program, based on what you learn over those three weeks. But I also want you to think about the goals that are more specific to you! What's your "why"—the reason that you personally want to complete the 21DSD? Will it mean that you've finally committed to doing something for yourself and followed through? Will it mean you've done something harder than you ever thought possible? Will it mean that you've supported a friend through the program? Changed some of the unhealthy habits your family had fallen into? Learned how to nourish your body so you feel good every day while eating healthy foods—and enjoyed it?!

Over the years that I've led folks through this program, I've learned this: once you complete the 21-Day Sugar Detox, your confidence level will spike. If you previously struggled with feeling incapable of doing things that are uncertain or scary for you, the positive effects of this program will go far beyond the physical. Yes, you'll absolutely feel great physically when you get rid of sugar, but the wave of pride that'll sweep over you when you successfully finish the 21DSD may be the exact boost you need to make some amazing changes in other areas of your life.

So now's the time to dig deep and uncover your goals for this program, your personal "why."

WHAT IS YOUR WHY?

Describe below, in as much detail as possible, the reason(s) why you want to break your sugar and carb cravings. What will it mean to you to complete this program? How will you feel when it's done—not only physically but also emotionally and mentally?

_____

_____

_____

_____

WHAT I ATE TODAY

B: _____   D: *Chicken Fajita Salad*

L: _____   S: _____

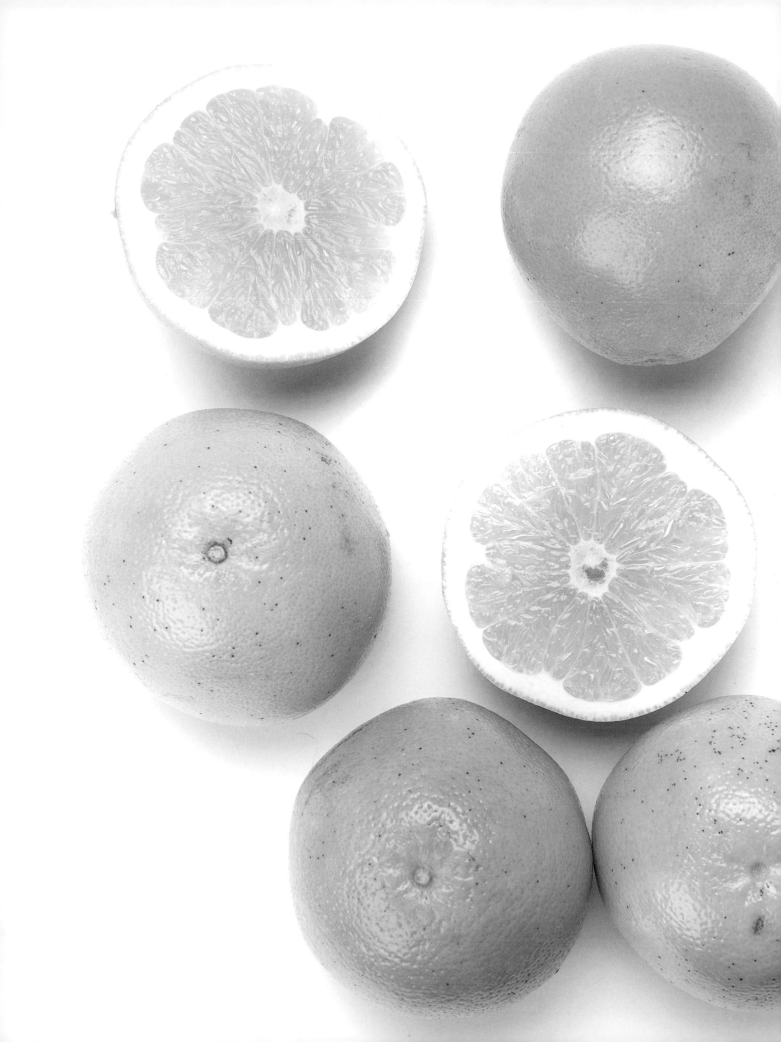

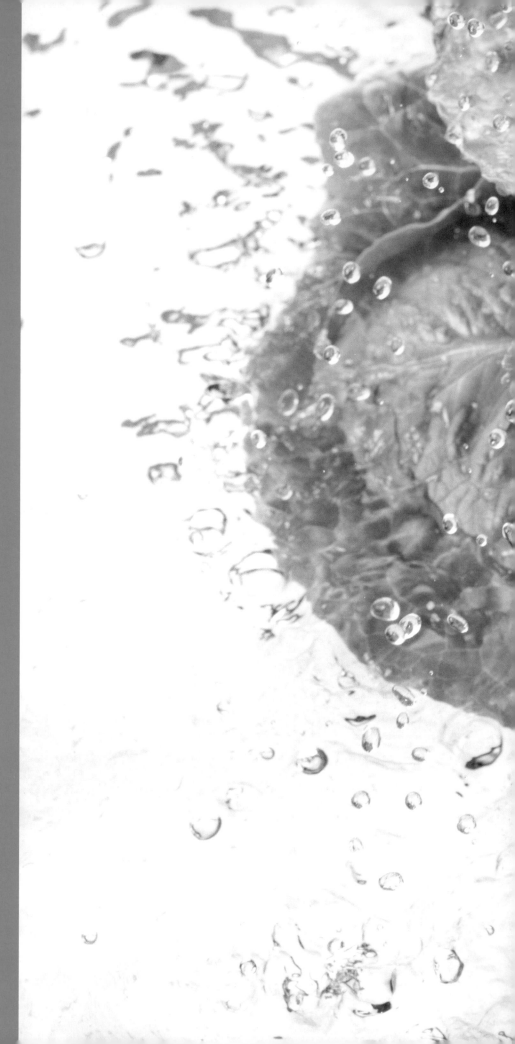

THE
21-DAY
SUGAR
DETOX

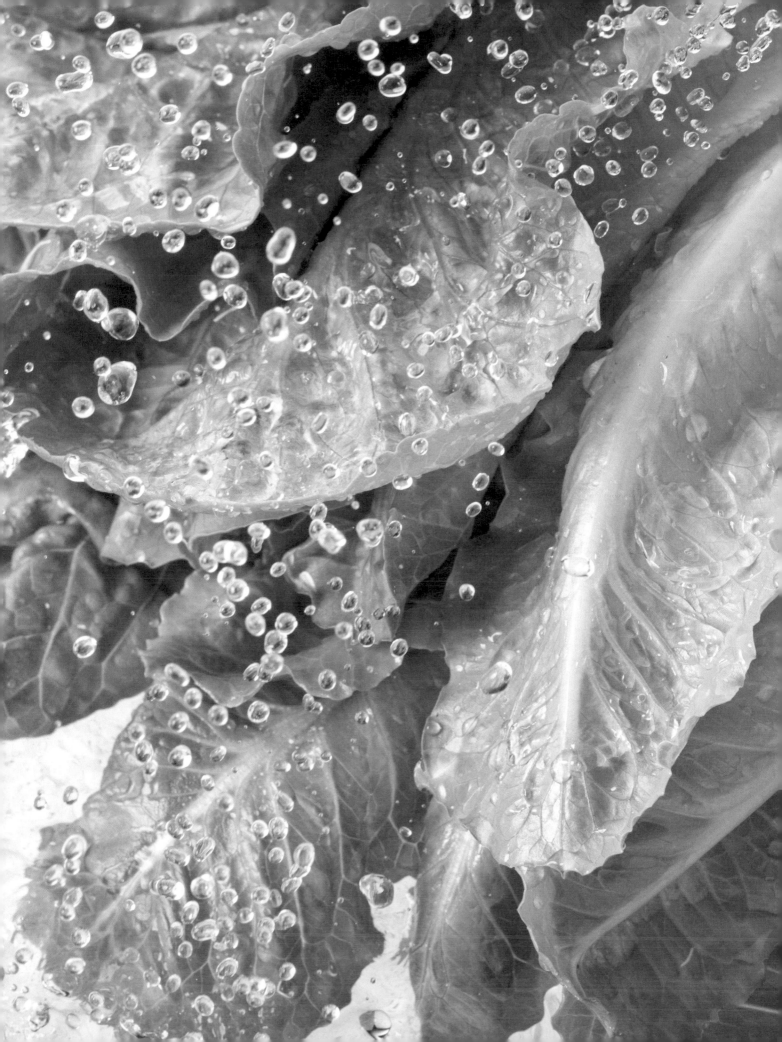

"I got this!"

You may experience: No effects at all, or possibly some extremely strong cravings later in the day. Those cravings are likely more emotional than physiological—your mind misses the foods you're not eating more than your body does at this point. You may feel extra hungry, or you may feel like you are eating a lot more food than you're used to—and that's okay! (Remember, this isn't a diet, so if you're hungry, eat something from the Yes foods list on page 20.)

Your best bet: Roll with the positivity that day 1 brings, and don't forget to eat the food you prepared!

The Dish from Diane

This is it! You're officially digging in, and I know you're feeling super prepared and ready for this. I want you to be present with yourself today. Feel what you're feeling and take notes about it in your journal. Are things all sunshine and rainbows? Or are you feeling a little nervous as you look ahead to the coming week? Shake off the nerves by getting into the kitchen and prepping some food, or by reaching out to your detox buddy or coach, or to the 21DSD community via social media. Remember, as we talked about during the pre-detox days, the key to success on the 21DSD is preparation, and second only to that is support. If you haven't yet reached out to connect with me, the 21-Day Sugar Detox community, or friends who are also doing the 21DSD, jump on it!

> **"One of the wonderful things about being alive is that it's never too late."**
>
> —Phyllis A. Whitney

DAY 1

TODAY'S LESSON
Foods that help you detox

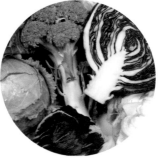

Did you know that your liver is one of the major powerhouses of your metabolism? It's responsible for filtering up to two quarts of blood each minute, clearing out toxins ranging from bacteria to chemical compounds like pharmaceutical drugs, alcohol, and pesticides. If your liver is healthy, it gets rid of nearly all toxins in a dual-phased process. Unfortunately, if it's not so healthy, detoxification can be dramatically impaired, creating a burden in your body that can manifest in a variety of symptoms, including poor digestion, fatigue, headaches, sensitivity to strong perfumes, fat-loss resistance, and hormonal imbalances. The liver also makes bile, which is a major player in breaking down and digesting fats.

Many people don't realize that in addition to its detoxification duties, the liver also helps manage blood sugar levels. So if your liver is overburdened with toxins and isn't in tip-top shape, blood sugar takes a hit.

Supporting your liver can be as simple as upping your intake of three delicious foods:

1. **Cruciferous veggies** (broccoli, cauliflower, cabbage, Brussels sprouts, kale, bok choy, radishes): Vitamin C, folate, and sulfur compounds in these are amazingly supportive for the liver, and the veggies add color and crunch to your plate.

2. **Avocado:** Rich in glutathione, a nutrient critical to completing both phases of liver detoxification—and a tasty source of healthy fats!

3. **Eggs:** The yolks are rich in choline, an amazing supporter for the liver. Eggs also give your liver the amino acids it needs to complete detoxification processes, so eat up!

Not sure how to get enough of these foods every day? Don't worry—simply following the meal plan in this guide (page 115) will get you there.

Allergic to eggs, or just or tired of them? Another great source of choline is liver! Look for organic and pastured sources to get the healthiest livers you can. If you're not a big fan of liver, try chicken livers—they have a milder flavor you won't even notice in recipes. Other 21DSD-friendly sources of choline include beef, salmon, and scallops.

TODAY'S MEALS

Breakfast:	Lunch:	Dinner:
Sausage, Spinach & Peppers Frittata (page 138)	*Leftover* Chicken Fajita Salad	Ranch Chicken & Bacon Stuffed Potatoes (page 166)

Snack(s): half an avocado + salsa with raw veggies

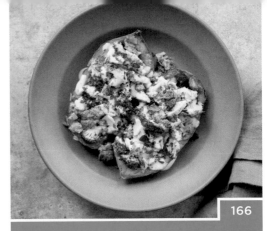

166

TODAY'S RECIPE
Ranch Chicken & Bacon Stuffed Potatoes

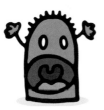

> HELLO, MY NAME IS HANGRY!

SHARE YOUR EXPERIENCE

Tag @21daysugardetox and use the hashtag #21DSD on Instagram. We'd love to see how you're doing!

TODAY'S CHECKLIST

- [ ] **Prep** Smoky Chicken Salad Lettuce Boats (page 172) for lunch days 2 & 4 and 4 slices bacon for lunch days 3 & 6.

- [ ] **Post to social media** using the hashtag #21DSD. Talk about your day 1 meals and experience—tell us your "why," what you're most excited about, and what your goal is for the program.

✏ NOTES ABOUT TODAY

A success I had today was... _____

_____

_____

_____

A challenging moment today was... _____

_____

_____

_____

Something that surprised me today was... _____

_____

_____

_____

notes _____

_____

SLEEP TIME & QUALITY

to bed last night _____

woke up today _____

- [ ] excellent
- [ ] fair
- [ ] good
- [ ] poor

EXERCISE

time _____

_____

type _____

_____

MOOD & ENERGY

- [ ] excellent
- [ ] fair
- [ ] good
- [ ] poor

TODAY'S FRUIT

🍎 or 🍌 or 🍊

WHAT TO EXPECT

*"This isn't so bad" or
"Will this get easier?!"*

You may experience: No symptoms at all, or you may be feeling it pretty intensely today with headaches, mental fogginess, or increased hunger.

Your best bet: Keep trucking! Make sure that your meals are well balanced and include enough protein and fat, along with the appropriate carbs for your activity level and your 21DSD plate (see pages 22–23).

The Dish from Diane

This is about the time when I typically see a lot of detoxers trying to "detox harder" or "really follow the rules" by not eating the recommended good carbs. I cannot stress this enough: you *cannot* make this program more effective by being more restrictive than the program dictates. By not eating your included fruit for the day, not adding extra carbs based on your activity level, or trying to eat the absolute bare minimum even if you're hungry, you do not make this program more successful—you just make it harder. It is already hard enough, and it is effective as written. And, ultimately, if you're more restrictive, you'll be far *less* successful. Not only will you want to quit the program because you'll feel terrible, but you're not truly helping yourself with this mindset and approach.

In fact, when you build a plate that includes more carbs each day, you will have much better success on the program. *Trust me.* You'll feel better in your workouts and you won't lose motivation to exercise because your energy will stay where you need it. Eating good-quality carbs fuels you well and keeps cravings at bay! So don't fear the fat, but also keep those carbs on your plate! That's how the 21DSD was designed.

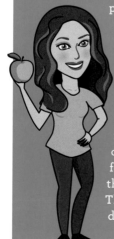

DAY 2

TODAY'S LESSON
Physically adjusting to the 21DSD

Some of the toughest days on this program tend to be days 3 through 7, a period during which many people experience "carb flu," or an energy dip, headaches, extra hunger and/or thirst, or even some weakness or a hint of a fever. Why not later in the program? You might think that the first week would be the easiest, and in a lot of ways, it is—your motivation is the highest, you're thinking more about preparation and planning, and the newness of it all is most exciting in week 1.

But week 1 can bring some of the biggest *physical* challenges, depending on how different your plate looks now. If you were eating a lot more carbs than your activity level required before you began the 21DSD, then days 3 through 7 are when things start to really change with your body.

Remember back to three days pre-detox (page 38) when we talked about glycogen, the carbohydrate stored in your liver and muscles? When you reduce the amount of carbs you consume, your body will start to dip into those glycogen stores, and a drop in the amount of stored glycogen largely accounts for the days when you feel the hit from the reduction in carb intake. As your body runs low on glycogen, you may feel a bit tired initially. (That energy will come back around days 7 through 10 as your body adapts to burning fat for fuel.)

Now, if your activity level means that you're eating more 21DSD-friendly starchy carbs (see page 20), then you may or may not experience this shift. If you're eating fewer good carbs because you're not very active or your daily activity is very low-intensity, it's likely going to hit you either tomorrow or on day 4.

You see, low-intensity activity—such as walking, lower-intensity weight lifting, yoga, or gardening—doesn't require much glycogen. In fact, these activities are very well fueled by dietary fat and by stored body fat. So your 21DSD plate of quality protein, plenty of veggies, and healthy fats will be perfect for you. Allow your body at least a week to adjust to this new balance of foods. While the adjustment may begin around day 3, it can last as long as a week or even two.

TODAY'S MEALS

Breakfast:
½ Banana Nut Smoothie + 2 hard-boiled eggs

Lunch:
Smoky Chicken Salad Lettuce Boats (page 172)

Dinner:
Leftover Ranch Chicken & Bacon Stuffed Potatoes

Snack(s): Smoky Toasted Nut Mix or jerky

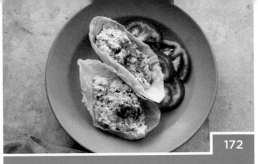

172

TODAY'S RECIPE
Smoky Chicken Salad Lettuce Boats

> ❝ *Day 2 and I'm feeling great! Actually pretty full after breakfast. Have been adding steamed spinach with a splash of lime on it to replace my morning toast and wow, what a difference in my sluggishness that makes! Had that with two egg muffins from the book and it was delicious and filling.* ❞
>
> — Joanna M. (21DSD Community Member)

TODAY'S CHECKLIST

- [ ] **Review your 21DSD plate** (pages 22–23) and be sure you're getting the good carbs you need.

- [ ] **Post to social media** using the hashtag #21DSD about your day 2 meals and experience. Tell us what kind of activity you have planned for your detox, whether it's walking, yoga, at-home workouts, CrossFit, or anything else!

✎ NOTES ABOUT TODAY

Today I was grateful for... _____

_____

_____

_____

Something I learned to stop doing was... _____

_____

_____

_____

Something I want to start doing is... _____

_____

_____

_____

notes _____

_____

SLEEP TIME & QUALITY

to bed last night _____

woke up today _____

- [ ] excellent   - [ ] fair
- [ ] good   - [ ] poor

EXERCISE

time _____

_____

type _____

_____

MOOD & ENERGY

- [ ] excellent   - [ ] fair
- [ ] good   - [ ] poor

TODAY'S FRUIT

🍎 or 🍌 or 🍊

WHAT TO EXPECT

"I think I've got this down."

You may experience: Fatigue, cold- and flu-like symptoms, low blood sugar, or self-doubt. Day 3 is the beginning of some of the hardest days for most folks!

Your best bet: Realize that you are likely not experiencing a real cold or flu but the effects of detoxing from sugar. Be careful not to rush off to the doctor; just know that this reaction is common and will subside within a few days. And if you're an active person, adding good carbs to your plate will likely squash these issues flat. Focus on the positives that are ahead—liberation from your cravings and a healthier you, inside and out.

The Dish from Diane

Today is a pretty big milestone! It's a day when a lot of folks throw in the towel, usually because they jumped in without preparing—but not you! You've been following along since the pre-detox week and you've got your eyes on the prize. Stay focused on each day as it comes, checking off your list for the day.

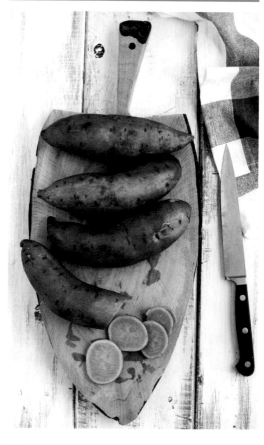

DAY 3

TODAY'S LESSON

Do you need more good carbs than you thought?

How are you feeling today? Are you starting to get the hang of the 21DSD after those first two days? Or are you still feeling like you're flailing a bit? Today's lesson is to help you figure out if perhaps you need more carbs than you originally thought you did.

Are you experiencing any of the following?

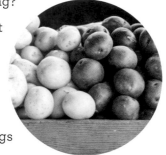

- Excessive fatigue (assuming you slept well the night before)

- Extreme hunger

- A headache that won't quit

- A feeling of general weakness or malaise when you exercise (or your legs feel like lead!)

If any of the above sounds like you, it may be time to revisit your 21DSD plate (pages 22–23)! I've often noticed that folks underestimate or undervalue how much activity they do while on the 21DSD. The more active you are, the more carbs you burn naturally in a day, so you can add them to your plate without concern that they'll keep your body from being able to *also* burn fat. If you have an active job where you're on your feet all or much of the day, if you are pregnant or nursing a little one, or if you're active in the gym or in sports during the day and you're feeling any of the symptoms listed above, you probably need a good-carb bump-up! This is normal and expected, and I encourage you to do it now before you get further into the program and feel these symptoms much more harshly.

"**Life is not merely to be alive, but to be well.**"

—Marcus Valerius Martialis

TODAY'S MEALS

Breakfast:	**Lunch:**	**Dinner:**
Leftover Sausage, Spinach & Peppers Frittata	Bacon, turkey, tomato, & avocado on lettuce leaves	Buffalo Cauliflower & Chicken Wings (page 162) + green salad

Snack(s): 21DSD Frozen Coco-Monkey Bites

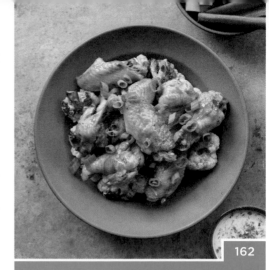

162

✎ NOTES ABOUT TODAY

I would describe today as...

_____

_____

_____

_____

Today I'm proud that...

_____

_____

_____

The most delicious thing I ate today was...

_____

_____

_____

notes _____

_____

_____

_____

_____

_____

_____

TODAY'S RECIPE
Buffalo Cauliflower & Chicken Wings

TODAY'S CHECKLIST

☐ **Post to social media** using the hashtag #21DSD about your day 3 meals and experience. Tell us how you plan to build your plate and what healthy carbs you're eating.

SLEEP TIME & QUALITY

to bed last night _____

woke up today _____

☐ excellent ☐ fair

☐ good ☐ poor

EXERCISE

time _____

_____

type _____

_____

MOOD & ENERGY

☐ excellent ☐ fair

☐ good ☐ poor

TODAY'S FRUIT

🍎 or 🍌 or 🍊

"Three days down, eighteen to go!"

You may experience: Mood changes, minor skin irritation, or breakouts. Acne is a common detox symptom and is a great sign that your body is working to clear toxins!

Your best bet: Remember that awareness is key when it comes to your mood. Try not to react to those around you in a hypersensitive way, and remember that the change in your diet is likely affecting your mood more than you realize. For your skin, add milk thistle (tea, tincture, or capsules) and ginger tea to aid in detoxification. Take care to read the list of ingredients in products you apply to your skin for ingredients that may cause further irritation, such as parabens (found in a variety of lotions, cosmetics, and cleansing products), sodium lauryl or laureth sulfate (often in shampoos and body washes, listed as SLS/SLES), and oxybenzone (often in sunscreens and moisturizers). If you're interested in switching to a safer, cleaner product, consider looking for one with charcoal in it for detox support, or check out the oil cleansing method, which uses natural oils to cleanse the skin instead of potentially irritating or harmful soaps.

The Dish from Diane

Day 4 brings unique challenges and can be a big turning point. It's often the beginning of some of the most uncomfortable days physically, but this is normal, and it *will* get better! Often people don't realize how big a change it is to stop eating sugar and unhealthy carbs, and how that can change how you feel so profoundly. As you adjust to this way of eating, remember that prepping meals and snacks about every three to four days is a good idea. So today may be your day to get some food ready for the rest of the week.

DAY 4

TODAY'S LESSON

Acne or skin rashes as a detox effect

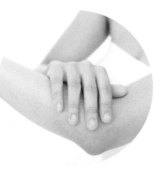

It's common to experience either an outbreak of acne or some light skin rashes around day 4 on the 21DSD. Exactly why this happens varies depending on the individual, but some common reasons include: a shift in blood sugar levels as they even out; a shift in the hormones your body produces as levels are beginning to balance out *or* because your liver function improves and toxins and/or hormones are being more efficiently flushed from your system; or a shift in gut bacteria and resulting digestive function changes. All of these changes are normal and expected, and detox-related acne and skin rashes should clear up pretty quickly. If they persist after your detox, I recommend that you consult your physician.

Now may be a great time to review some of your skincare products as an extension of your detox. You certainly don't need to do this to complete the 21DSD, but it's a good reminder to examine how what you put on our skin is impacting your health. I recommend going to the Environmental Working Group's Skin Deep website (ewg.org/skindeep) and searching their database for the products you use—they have a ton of information on ingredients in common skincare products and potential health concerns. You can also search the site for some safer, healthier options for skincare products.

> **"There are two ways to face the future. One way is with apprehension; the other is with anticipation."**
>
> —Jim Rohn

TODAY'S MEALS

Breakfast:
Breakfast Salad (page 130)

Lunch:
Leftover Smoky Chicken Salad Lettuce Boats

Dinner:
Grilled steak (see page 116) + Crispy Brussels Sprouts (page 194)

Snack(s): 21DSD Frozen Coco-Monkey Bites

> ❝ *I had a headache on days 4 and 5 . . . Day 4 was pretty gnarly but day 5 wasn't as bad. I've definitely had mood swings, but those were the worst on day 3. I'm hoping these effects subside pretty soon!*
>
> *I'm very surprised that I haven't had any cravings, although I somewhat feel like a drug addict going through withdrawals. It will pass. Other than that I feel great! Not as hungry in the last few days as the first, but it tends to fluctuate. I've really been enjoying the food I've been making!* ❞
>
> — Jessica B. (21DSD Community Member)

✎ NOTES ABOUT TODAY

Right now, the 21DSD is difficult in that... _____

_____

_____

_____

What's made life easier has been... _____

_____

_____

_____

Physically and emotionally, I'm feeling... _____

_____

_____

_____

notes _____

_____

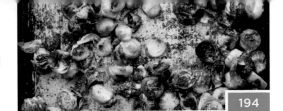

194

TODAY'S RECIPE
Crispy Brussels Sprouts

TODAY'S CHECKLIST

☐ **Review your skincare routine.** If you're struggling with acne or rashes, it may be from the detox, but you may also want to try new skincare options.

☐ **Prep** Bacon, Brussels, Asparagus & Goat Cheese Frittata (page 140) for breakfast days 6 & 7.

☐ **Prep** 2 small sweet potatoes for dinner day 6 and lunch day 8.

☐ **Post to social media** using the hashtag #21DSD about your day 4 meals and experience. Tell us what other parts of your life are being influenced by your newfound healthy outlook.

SLEEP TIME & QUALITY

to bed last night _____

woke up today _____

☐ excellent ☐ fair

☐ good ☐ poor

EXERCISE

time _____

type _____

MOOD & ENERGY

☐ excellent ☐ fair

☐ good ☐ poor

TODAY'S FRUIT

🍎 or 🍌 or 🍊

"Okay, I'm getting the hang of this!"

You may experience: Fewer headaches and fewer cravings, or struggles with temptation and slipups if you're unprepared and hunger sets in.

Your best bet: Remember what got you off on the right foot in the first place: preparation! You were right on in getting food ready, having healthy snacks on hand, and planning meals, and now you may need to revisit that preparation. Or, as the weekend approaches, follow the tips in today's lesson to get ready for dining out for the first time.

The Dish from Diane

Dining out may initially seem daunting on the 21DSD, but it's an amazing opportunity! What I love about having three full weeks on this program is that you'll inevitably be faced with normal life circumstances, like dining out, and you'll learn a new way to navigate them. This is one big reason why this program isn't much shorter—so that you don't simply have a way to eat while on the 21DSD but learn and become used to making healthier choices for the long term. So use your dining-out experience as a time to learn. If you're headed to a restaurant you go to often, it's a great time to reevaluate your old favorites—find a new way to put a plate together by ordering something a bit more customized. If it's a new place you've never been to before, use the tips from today to get on the right path.

A common stumbling block is worrying about eating an off-program food or ingredient by accident at a restaurant. Sometimes ingredients sneak into sauces or dressings, or even soups, stews, and so on. If you think you may have inadvertently eaten something off-plan, just keep moving forward.

DAY 5

TODAY'S LESSON
Dining out on the 21DSD

Things may seem to be going really smoothly now, until you start thinking about the weekend and how you may not be eating at home for a change. Here are some tips to keep you on track when dining out, 21DSD-style!

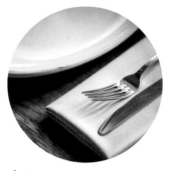

1. Know before you go! Preview the restaurant's menu online before you go. While some restaurants are slow to update their website as the menu changes, most are fairly consistent, and even if the menu has changed, they'll have something you can easily select after your preview. This is also a great time to read reviews from other diners on a site like Yelp, OpenTable, or TripAdvisor to see how accommodating a restaurant may be to making requested modifications to a dish.

2. Don't arrive starving. Before you head out the door, eat a small snack of some nuts or nut butter, half of an avocado, or some leftover protein.

3. Pass on the bread basket. If your companions are eating bread and the temptation gets to be too much, ask for sliced veggies or olives to nibble on.

4. Skip the appetizers or opt for a salad starter. It's often tough to find 21DSD-friendly appetizers, though there are some! Antipasto, oysters, shrimp cocktail, and chicken skewers may work, but you're better off focusing on your main dish. If your friends are getting apps and you want to start eating at the same time, order a green salad with olive oil and lemon or vinegar as a dressing. Remember that a lot of premade salad dressings contain not only sugars but unhealthy oils—stick to olive oil!

5. Ask questions about entrées. While finger food is often breaded, fried, or otherwise carb-loaded, entrées made of simpler ingredients can be easy to find. Look for grilled, broiled, or baked options, which are usually safer bets for 21DSD dining. But ask the server for details on how things are prepared; they're used to questions! Be polite, but get the answers you need.

6. Make substitutions. If a meal comes with french fries, bread, or pasta, ask that the kitchen leave it off of the plate, or substitute some vegetables or a baked potato or sweet potato (if your 21DSD plate calls for it) instead.

TODAY'S MEALS

Breakfast:
½ Banana Nut Smoothie + 2 hard-boiled eggs

Lunch:
Leftover Buffalo Cauliflower & Chicken Wings + green salad

Dinner:
½ *batch* Super Garlic Salmon & Vegetables (page 188)

Snack(s): Smoky Toasted Nut Mix or jerky

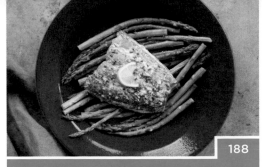

188

TODAY'S RECIPE
Super Garlic Salmon & Vegetables

TODAY'S CHECKLIST

☐ **Review the Guide to Dining Out (page 108).** This will give you the heads-up on some easy 21DSD choices in several types of cuisines.

☐ **Post to social media** using the hashtag #21DSD about your day 5 meals and experience. If you dined out, show us what you picked from the menu!

> "Acknowledging a mistake just means that you are wiser today than you were yesterday."
>
> —Kelly Ann Rothaus

NOTES ABOUT TODAY

A few local restaurants I can dine at on the 21DSD are...
_____
_____
_____

What I can order from the menu (maybe with a tweak) is...
_____
_____
_____

Some restaurants I'll avoid for the 21DSD are...
_____
_____
_____

notes_____
_____

SLEEP TIME & QUALITY
to bed last night _____
woke up today _____

☐ excellent   ☐ fair
☐ good   ☐ poor

EXERCISE
time _____
_____
type _____
_____

MOOD & ENERGY
☐ excellent   ☐ fair
☐ good   ☐ poor

TODAY'S FRUIT
🍎 or 🍌 or 🍊

WHAT TO EXPECT

"How can I make week 2 as successful as week 1?"

You may experience: Cold- or flu-like symptoms beginning to subside.

Your best bet: Stay on track with your daily checklist and meal plan details to be sure that you are ready for week 2 before it starts.

The Dish from Diane

Sticking to healthy habits while traveling can often make you feel like an oddball, especially if you're away from home for work and your coworkers couldn't care less about healthy eating choices. Often, travel is seen as a time to let your hair down, unwind, and not try to maintain squeaky-clean eating habits. But when you're on the 21DSD, you're committed. And if you're traveling for work, then this isn't a vacation! It's another workday, and treating it as a vacation and a reason to break your commitment to the 21DSD won't serve you in any positive way.

Some popular hotel chains that have kitchens include: Embassy Suites, Extended Stay America, Home2 Suites by Hilton, Homewood Suites, Hyatt House, Hyatt Summerfield Suites, Residence Inn by Marriott, Springhill Suites, and Staybridge Suites by Marriott.

You can also look for chains whose name includes the word "suites" or "extended stay"—those will have kitchens as well.

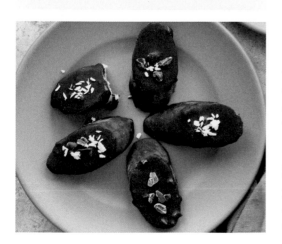

DAY 6

TODAY'S LESSON
Traveling 21DSD style

While I don't recommend you tackle a 21DSD over a family vacation, having a work trip or frequent travel for business isn't a reason not to complete the detox. Work travel is part of your everyday life, so learning how to make healthy choices when you travel is a good idea.

To stay on track, whether you're home or away, requires (1) forethought, (2) commitment, and (3) follow-through. But at home, you have the ease and comfort of your own kitchen, and it's easier to control everything, from where you shop to how you cook your food to the time you eat. Here are some practical tips for making your traveling 21DSD easier.

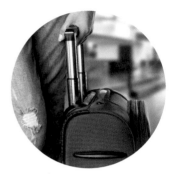

Prep or buy travel snacks ahead of time. Jerky, meat sticks, or pork chicharrones/cracklings; nut butter, coconut butter, or seed butter packets; homemade trail mix or nuts; cut veggies with single-serving guacamole packets; and small servings of cheese (for Levels 1 and 2) are great snack options.

Book a hotel room with a kitchen. Lots of hotels offer extended-stay-style rooms with a full-sized refrigerator, a burner or two, plates, glasses, pots and pans, a dishwasher, and a coffeepot. Some even have food storage containers for leftovers! If you're booking your own room or can make this request, do it! If you aren't booking the travel and are stuck with a room that doesn't offer these amenities, then simply call ahead to ask that a mini fridge be in your room when you arrive (see the next tip).

Request a mini fridge. All hotels have mini fridges handy in case a guest needs to keep medications cool. If the hotel asks why you need a mini fridge when you request it, you can say that you have specific dietary requirements, but they likely won't ask. It's more common now for hotel rooms to have a mini fridge by default, though many are stocked with alcohol or treats—simply remove those or ask housekeeping to remove them. You can also ask that they be removed ahead of your stay. Trust me, the hotel is in the business of accommodating your needs—ask for what you want and they'll help out.

Identify a local grocery store before you hit the road. When you arrive, time permitting, head to the grocery store before you do anything else. Simply unload your bags and head out to stock up on some items. This plan may involve adjusting your flight time to allow time to go to the store before your first appointment or meeting. Again, if you are in charge of these decisions, make them accordingly. If there's a travel department or person booking your flights, request that you arrive earlier in the day. Remember, you don't get what you don't ask for, so it's always worth the request!

Prepare breakfast in your room. Whether you bring hard-boiled eggs from home or simply eat ready-made foods that are 21DSD-friendly (for instance, some deli meats or a green apple with nut butter), having breakfast ready to go is a huge help when away from home. If you've got a breakfast meeting, it's easy enough to order some poached eggs with bacon and some vegetables for your meal.

TODAY'S MEALS

Breakfast:	Lunch:	Dinner:
Bacon, Brussels, Asparagus & Goat Cheese Frittata (page 140)	Bacon, turkey, tomato, & avocado on lettuce leaves	Cheesesteak Stuffed Potatoes (page 168)

Snack(s): 21DSD Frozen Coco-Monkey Bites

NOTES ABOUT TODAY

What helped me stay focused today was... _____

_____

_____

_____

Something that could have derailed me was... _____

_____

_____

_____

I'm preparing for the next couple of days by... _____

_____

_____

_____

notes _____

_____

_____

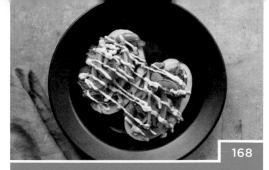

168

TODAY'S RECIPE
Cheesesteak Stuffed Potatoes

TODAY'S CHECKLIST

☐ **Traveling 21DSD-style?** Do your research and make a list of places you can eat, nearby grocery stores, and what you need to prep for the trip.

☐ **Prep** 21DSD Ketchup (page 232) and Smoky Toasted Nut Mix (page 212) for snacks.

☐ **Post to social media** using the hashtag #21DSD about your day 6 meals and experience. If you travel on the 21DSD, show us how you roll!

SLEEP TIME & QUALITY

to bed last night _____

woke up today _____

☐ excellent ☐ fair

☐ good ☐ poor

EXERCISE

time _____

_____

type _____

_____

MOOD & ENERGY

☐ excellent ☐ fair

☐ good ☐ poor

TODAY'S FRUIT

🍎 or 🍌 or 🍊

The Dish from Diane

Do not, I repeat, do not throw in the towel after one week! The weekends tend to be some of the toughest days. Facing social events, dining out, friends who aren't on the 21DSD with you ... The list of reasons why this can get rocky goes on and on. Be here now. Be present with yourself, and yank yourself out of the downward spiral of a headspace that tells you to quit. I know it gets hard. But you knew this wasn't going to be easy, right? Now's the time to revisit your "why." Why did you start? You know that if you hang with me for the full three weeks, what awaits you on the other side is not only a newfound set of skills and feeling better physically, but a new sense of confidence that, yes, you can do hard things. And, yes, you are capable and strong—and while situations that challenge you will come along, they won't shake you. You've got this!

> **"If you do nothing unexpected, nothing unexpected happens."**
>
> —Fay Weldon

DAY 7

TODAY'S LESSON
All this grocery shopping— how can I save money?!

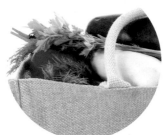

Here's the hard truth: your grocery bill may increase while you complete this program. The reality here is that stocking your house (especially your pantry, initially) does add up. Unfortunately, fresh meats, seafood, eggs, and vegetables don't benefit from the government subsidies that make processed foods a lot less expensive. Plus, the way the cost of groceries balances out to the rest of your budget is something you're currently not used to. What I mean is, the dollars you spend on healthy food have a direct effect on health and wellness. The more your health improves because you're eating high-quality, nutrient-dense foods (and, just as important, because you're not eating foods high in sugar), the less you'll spend on things like pain medications, cold care, doctors' visits, and beyond.

Choosing to spend more on healthy foods means a major shift in lifestyle and priorities. That said, there *are* ways to make healthy shopping and eating more budget-friendly. Here are my best tips!

Spend more on healthy fats and proteins. Whenever you can grab organic fats and oils (like coconut oil and olive oil, for example), it's a good idea to do so.

How to save on healthy fats and proteins:

- Make ghee at home from grass-fed butter—I promise, it's super easy. (See the recipe on page 247.) You'll save a lot over buying premade versions, and your house will smell great while you make it!

- Buy meat in bulk and on sale. Stocking up on proteins at a bulk rate or when they're on sale is very budget-friendly if you have some space to freeze them. A basic chest freezer (provided you have a bit of space in a garage or storage area with power) runs about $150 or less and will save you a ton in the long term! Of course, you can also freeze extra protein in your regular freezer, especially once the ice cream has been kicked out (wink). Consider buying meat in bulk from a local rancher or farmer—find one in your area on eatwild.com.

Spend less on healthy carbs like vegetables, 21DSD-friendly fruits, and, for Level 1, gluten-free grains. When buying produce, go for local and organic as often as you can, but don't sweat it if you need to mix it up with conventionally grown produce.

How to save on healthy carbs:

- Buying in season is almost always more affordable. There are lots of guides to in-season produce online, and it may be a good idea to print one out and hang it on your fridge so it's handy when you're planning meals and swaps.

- Bulk gluten-free grains are a really great budget solution. Many grocery stores either have bins or larger bags of gluten-free grains that cost less per pound. Whenever possible, get these without packaging from bulk bins—that'll save you the most.

TODAY'S MEALS

Breakfast:	Lunch:	Dinner:
Leftover Bacon, Brussels, Asparagus & Goat Cheese Frittata	*½ batch* Super Garlic Salmon & Vegetables (page 188)	Tangy Chicken Salad (page 176)

Snack(s): 21DSD Frozen Coco-Monkey Bites

✏ NOTES ABOUT TODAY

The best thing I did for myself this week was... _____

_____

_____

_____

A challenge I overcame this weekend was... _____

_____

_____

_____

One goal I have for next week is... _____

_____

_____

_____

notes _____

_____

_____

176

TODAY'S RECIPE
Tangy Chicken Salad

TODAY'S CHECKLIST

☐ **Revisit your "why."** Spend time journaling at least a few sentences about why you started on this journey.

☐ **Prep** Pumpkin Spice Smoothie (page 145) and hard-boil 6 eggs for breakfast days 8, 9 & 11.

☐ **Prep** 21DSD Cinnamon Banana Bread (page 220) for snacks.

☐ **Prep** sauces and condiments per the meal plan on page 117.

☐ **Post to social media** using the hashtag #21DSD about your day 7 meals and experience. If you have a great budget tip, share it with us!

SLEEP TIME & QUALITY

to bed last night _____

woke up today _____

☐ excellent   ☐ fair

☐ good   ☐ poor

EXERCISE

time _____

_____

type _____

_____

MOOD & ENERGY

☐ excellent   ☐ fair

☐ good   ☐ poor

TODAY'S FRUIT

🍎 or 🍌 or 🍊

"Wow, almost a whole week down. I feel awesome! But my digestion, not so much!"

You may experience: Digestive issues such as bloating, constipation, or diarrhea. These symptoms may be discouraging, but there's hope!

Your best bet: Follow the advice given today. We've got your digestion covered!

The Dish from Diane

"I'm experiencing some not-so-pleasant effects from these healthy dietary changes. Diane, what gives?!"

I hear you. It seems backward that you might physically experience something negative when you're eating healthier foods! How can that be?! Well, our bodies are really great at adapting to whatever it is we're doing, but that's not always a good thing. When we eat unhealthy food for a long time, our bodies get used to it, and in the short term, eating high-quality, nutrient-dense foods can cause it to scramble to adapt to the new, healthier input. And often it does take more than three weeks for your digestion to find a new normal when you ditch the highly processed carbs that were feeding your gut bacteria in a different way.

For many people, this change is miraculous and only has positive effects! But for others, this stage in the detox may make you question your decision to take it on. Heed today's advice and I promise things will regulate again before you know it!

> **"Difficulties mastered are opportunities won."**
>
> — Winston Churchill

DAY 8

TODAY'S LESSON
Digestion in question

Digestion is a hot topic on a 21DSD! I would be remiss if I didn't tackle this sensitive subject, since it's very likely that you'll run into some ups and downs over the course of this program. While many people don't experience any disruption at all during the program, it is common that issues happen.

The two most common digestive concerns that can arise on the 21DSD are:

1. a serious "back up" (aka constipation)
2. "everybody out" (aka diarrhea or loose stools)

These changes are the result of an increase in insoluble fiber from vegetables and a decrease in simple sugars (from the refined carbs you've eliminated), along with shifts in your hydration—reducing carb intake means that you need to drink more water to maintain hydration.

I know it's tough to read about this in the middle of some pep talks about your program and cozied up next to references to some yummy recipes, but bear with me! Now is the time when these issues tend to crop up, and I'd like to make sure you're equipped with the tools you need to best handle them.

Tips for handling constipation

- Add fermented foods like raw sauerkraut, kombucha, or fermented pickles to your daily meals. Note that all of these are sold in the refrigerated section of grocery stores.

- Include foods that contain soluble fiber, such as carrots, beets, parsnips, butternut squash, and sweet potatoes, in at least two meals per day.

- Include foods that contain prebiotic fiber, such as asparagus, jicama, artichokes, onions, and garlic.

- In at least one meal per day, include foods that contain resistant starches, such as a green-tipped banana or white potatoes that have been cooked and then cooled (all levels), or brown rice or legumes that have been cooked and then cooled (Level 1). Cooling these foods after cooking increases their gut bacteria–friendly nature, encouraging improved digestive function. Note that cooked-and-cooled starches can be reheated before eating to receive the same benefit.

All of the above will help to support a healthy balance of bacteria in the gut and promote more regular bowel movements.

Tips for handling diarrhea or loose stools

- Add a cup or more per day of bone broth. It can be sipped alone or consumed in soup or slow-cooked foods.
- Drink herbal, peppermint, chamomile, or ginger tea.
- Add fermented foods like raw sauerkraut, kombucha, or fermented pickles to your daily meals. Note that all of these are sold in the refrigerated section of grocery stores.
- Eat fennel or fennel seeds with or after meals. Raw is okay.
- Consider supplementing with L-glutamine and a high-quality probiotic that contains acidophilus.
- Avoid leafy greens, like kale and collards—eat more cooked foods than raw salads.
- Avoid nuts, seeds, and legumes (even if you're Level 1).

All of the above will help to heal an irritated digestive system. Start with the steps that are easiest for you, see how you feel, and go from there.

Your digestion may be moving along perfectly, and if so, great! But if you are experiencing constipation or diarrhea, don't worry; these changes in digestive function are common and to be expected when the food on your plate every day changes. The more different your 21DSD food is from what you were eating prior to the program, the more it may impact your gut. But rest assured, the foods included in this program contribute plenty of healthy carbohydrates, fats, and fiber to keep your digestive system moving properly! Sometimes you just need to make a few small changes to get yourself back on track.

TODAY'S MEALS

Breakfast:	Lunch:	Dinner:
⅓ Pumpkin Spice Smoothie + 2 hard-boiled eggs	*Leftover* Cheesesteak Stuffed Potatoes	Grilled Pork Fall Salad (page 182)

Snack(s): Smoky Toasted Nut Mix or jerky

✎ NOTES ABOUT TODAY

My digestion so far has felt... _____

_____

_____

How I'll change or maintain that is by... _____

_____

_____

A new favorite food I've discovered is... _____

_____

_____

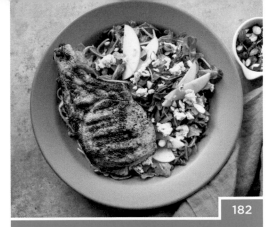

182

TODAY'S RECIPE
Grilled Pork Fall Salad

TODAY'S CHECKLIST

☐ **Address your digestion.** If things don't feel normal, take the steps in today's lesson to remedy it!

☐ **Post to social media** using the hashtag #21DSD about your day 8 meals. If you've got a tip for others on what got you through week 1, share it!

SLEEP TIME & QUALITY

to bed last night _____

woke up today _____

☐ excellent   ☐ fair

☐ good   ☐ poor

EXERCISE

time _____

_____

type _____

_____

MOOD & ENERGY

☐ excellent   ☐ fair

☐ good   ☐ poor

TODAY'S FRUIT

🍎 or 🍌 or 🍊

"I'm getting tired of the food I'm eating!"

You may experience: Feeling overwhelmed by how much time is involved in food prep.

Your best bet: Remember that there are tons of easy recipes right here in this book, and if these aren't perfect for you, there are countless 21DSD-friendly recipes online and in *The 21-Day Sugar Detox* and *The 21-Day Sugar Detox Cookbook*. Visit 21DSD.com for even more resources and links!

The Dish from Diane

When you decide to make changes in your life, there will always be some objectors or naysayers. Heck, even people who are very close to you may try to bring you down. Dig your heels in! You've got this, and the reason you decided to tackle the 21DSD has nothing to do with them—so don't let them get in your way. Are they in your body every day, feeling what you feel? No. No one else is responsible for the way you choose to live your life, not even someone you share your life with, like your spouse. Your choices are solely your own, and you get to make them as you need to. You're a capable adult, and you're doing what's best for you for three weeks. Remember, you don't need anyone's approval to decide to make positive changes in your own life—you only need to decide for yourself that it's what you want, then make it happen.

> "What we do today, right now, will have an accumulated effect on all our tomorrows."
>
> — Alexandra Stoddard

DAY 9

TODAY'S LESSON
Unsupportive friends and family

Not everyone will support your decision to do the 21-Day Sugar Detox, and the lack of support can turn otherwise fun occasions, from holiday get-togethers to office parties, into stressful events. When you're faced with critical friends or family members, it's important to consider the reason behind their lack of support.

Whether it's a well-meaning grandmother, a curious but skeptical coworker, a disappointed parent, a vegan or vegetarian uncle, a doctor cousin, or even your best buddy who's been with you since your beer-and-pizza days, there's always an underlying, more complete reason for their lack of support. Once you identify the reason behind their disapproval, you can plan how to handle your interactions with this person going forward. For a lot more on this, review pages 29 to 30 on strategies for handling other people's thoughts and feelings.

Some quick tips for dealing with unsupportive friends and family:

1. Keep your mindset positive and avoid complaining about tough moments during your detox.

2. Be proactive in as many situations as possible, such as selecting the restaurant where you'll dine out together.

3. Focus on your "why" and your own goals for completing the 21DSD.

4. Remind them that your desire to make these changes is only about you, not about them, and that you aren't asking them to make the same changes.

5. Deflect conversations that may become critical of your choices, and if it comes up, quickly change the subject to something less heated or emotional.

6. Avoid commenting on their choices (particularly around food) so that you're not encouraging this type of communication between you.

7. Set yourself up for success with support and accountability outside of the unsupportive network.

TODAY'S MEALS

Breakfast:	Lunch:	Dinner:
⅓ Pumpkin Spice Smoothie + 2 hard-boiled eggs	*Leftover* Tangy Chicken Salad	BBQ Burgers with Spicy Slaw (page 154)

Snack(s): 2 slices 21DSD Cinnamon Banana Bread + nut butter

154

❝ *This may be a bit more info than you want to know, but I'm super excited that my hot flashes have completely disappeared!!! I used to get them multiple times a day (and during the night). I'm on day 9 of the detox and noticed a few days ago that they had completely disappeared. Another great side effect of the 21DSD! Woo Hoo!* **❞**

— Lisa S. (21DSD Community Member)

✎ NOTES ABOUT TODAY

Time for a refresher: my "why" is... _____

_____

_____

_____

A time when I was able to easily explain why I'm doing the 21DSD was...

_____

_____

_____

A recipe I've made that I'll add to my regular rotation is... _____

_____

_____

_____

notes _____

_____

TODAY'S CHECKLIST

☐ **Prepare your script.** If people around you aren't supportive, be ready with your script! See pages 28-30 for simple ways to handle these scenarios.

☐ **Prep Slow Cooker BBQ Pulled Pork** (page 158) for dinner days 10, 17 & 19.

☐ **Post to social media** using the hashtag #21DSD about your day 9 meals. If you've got a tip for others on how you handle the naysayers, share it!

SLEEP TIME & QUALITY

to bed last night _____

woke up today _____

☐ excellent ☐ fair

☐ good ☐ poor

EXERCISE

time _____

_____

type _____

_____

MOOD & ENERGY

☐ excellent ☐ fair

☐ good ☐ poor

TODAY'S FRUIT

🍎 or 🍌 or 🍊

You may experience: If you had digestive issues such as gas and bloating, they're clearing up. You're getting into the swing of cooking, and you have collected a bunch of recipes to try.

Your best bet: Make some new shopping lists and try a new recipe! If you neglected shopping and food prep during week 1, get back into it now. If you were following the meal plan but realized your tastes are just different, plan some other meals for yourself!

The Dish from Diane

It's popular right now to follow an eating plan that dictates the exact number of grams of fat, protein, and carbs going into your body each day. And while that approach does hold some merit in the grand scheme of things—we can't escape the fact that, at some point, how much we eat does matter!—it certainly isn't the whole story. In fact, I'd argue that while "counting macros" is suitable in the short term and is helpful for specific body-fat manipulation goals, for long-term health and well-being (as well as a balanced state of mind and learning how to eat more intuitively), it tends to fail. Why? Well, when you get really hung up on the numbers, you lose the sense of self-reliance that's necessary to sustain healthy habits in the long-term. The 21DSD is about learning to make better food choices based on nutrient density and tuning in to your body's appetite cues, so you can eat what and how much your body needs, not what and how much a plan dictates. Inevitably, a rigid approach to long-term nutrition isn't sustainable, so I want you to learn to make healthy choices in a balance that works for you more than I want you to count or measure anything specifically.

DAY 10

TODAY'S LESSON
Nutrient density: Why real food matters more than calories

Eating whole, nutrient-dense sources of carbohydrates, like vegetables, fruits, roots, and tubers, enables you to make nutritional deposits into your body's "energy bank account." Sugar, however, which is empty of nutrients, asks your body for a withdrawal without making a deposit in return.

Let me explain what that means. To metabolize carbohydrates and turn them into energy, your body needs B vitamins and the minerals phosphorus, magnesium, iron, copper, manganese, zinc, and chromium. Bad carbs—refined, processed, and nutrient-poor—don't contain those vitamins and minerals in naturally occurring forms. So to process those carbs, your body has to use nutrients it already has stored. In other words, you have to make a withdrawal from your energy bank account. Nutrients are being used up, and no new nutrients are being provided. While we do get energy from calories, in order to turn the calories into energy, we need nutrients for that process to happen. So, calories without nutrients will only get you so far in creating cellular energy.

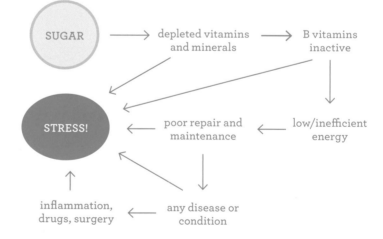

Low nutrient density explains why a diet rich in bad carbs leaves you feeling tired and often depleted of energy. It's also why you feel hungry more often—because your body is telling you to eat more food to get more nutrients! It doesn't want you to eat more nutrient-poor bad carbs; it's begging you to eat good stuff loaded with vitamins and minerals to satisfy that need for micronutrients at the cellular level. The problem is, what's most readily available usually isn't the good stuff—unless you plan ahead!

TODAY'S MEALS

Breakfast:
Breakfast Salad (page 130)

Lunch:
Leftover BBQ Burgers with Spicy Slaw

Dinner:
BBQ Pulled Pork Tacos with Spicy Slaw (page 158)

Snack(s): Smoky Toasted Nut Mix or jerky

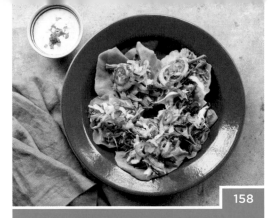

158

TODAY'S RECIPE
BBQ Pulled Pork Tacos with Spicy Slaw

✏ NOTES ABOUT TODAY

A nutrient-poor food I'll replace with a nutrient-dense one is...

_____
_____
_____
_____

I know that eating nutrient-dense food is important because...

_____
_____
_____
_____
_____
_____
_____

A success I had today was... _____

_____
_____
_____
_____
_____

notes _____

_____
_____
_____
_____

TODAY'S CHECKLIST

☐ **Freeze** ½ batch Slow Cooker BBQ Pulled Pork.

☐ **Post to social media** using the hashtag #21DSD about your day 10 experience and share what you'll use to replace nutrient-poor refined foods like bread or cereal.

SLEEP TIME & QUALITY

to bed last night _____

woke up today _____

☐ excellent   ☐ fair

☐ good   ☐ poor

EXERCISE

time _____

_____

type _____

_____

MOOD & ENERGY

☐ excellent   ☐ fair

☐ good   ☐ poor

TODAY'S FRUIT

🍎 or 🍌 or 🍊

You may experience: An acute awareness of how food was making you feel before the 21DSD; surprise that you aren't noticing many cravings anymore.

Your best bet: Make some notes about how you're feeling and recount to yourself some of the struggles and successes you've experienced. Reflect on the first ten days of your 21DSD journal and note where you've made changes and small successes along the way!

The Dish from Diane

Okay, I'm going to level with you today, because you're about halfway through this program and I don't want you getting through the second half and feeling as if you failed at anything. Here it is: all of your cravings *may not disappear* in three weeks. Yikes. I'm sorry.

Here's the thing: Only consuming high-quality food during the program will help free you from physical cravings for carbs and sugar. That's a big win right there. But for many, *emotional* cravings are even stronger. And tackling the reasons why we reach for food in a moment of sadness or stress, well, that can take a little more time.

But the longer you eat real, whole foods, the easier it becomes not to rely on sweets for a temporary little happiness boost. Yes, you will still eat sweet foods after the 21DSD, but you won't feel compelled to, unable to say no and pulled in so strongly that you almost don't realize what you're doing until you've eaten half a dozen cookies.

"Do what you can, with what you have, where you are."

— Theodore Roosevelt

DAY 11

TODAY'S LESSON
My cravings are gone. But *how*?!

Cravings have two components: (1) the emotional and (2) the physical. With this program, you change your body's physical responses to food by only allowing the really good-quality stuff into your body, and that means your physical cravings for carbs and sugar get better. Emotional cravings are a little trickier.

Stress and emotional triggers vary from person to person, and how we handle them also varies. You're here with us on this detox, so chances are, one of your ways of handling stress has been to reach for something sweet or carby. I get it. It's so common, and there's a real scientific basis for it.

The neurotransmitters serotonin and dopamine are responsible for feelings of either calm and happiness or compulsion and anxiety. Since eating carbs can trigger the release of both, when either serotonin or dopamine are low, the urge to grab sweets is increased. I probably didn't need to remind you of that, right? It's a familiar experience: feel stress or even sadness, reach for sweets or junky carbs, feel better (at least temporarily).

But you've just spent the last ten days *not* reaching for sugar or poor-quality carbs! You've been forcing yourself to find other means of feeling good—eating better-quality food, cooking, going for a walk, taking an extra yoga class, or calling (or texting, because who are we kidding) a friend. In short, you're replacing the act of eating sugar or carbs with healthier habits. And as you do so, those cravings are starting to disappear.

Furthermore, there's an additional phenomenon that hundreds of thousands of 21DSD participants have reported happening to them: *you crave what you eat.*

That means that the more you eat healthy foods, the more you'll crave those healthy foods. And those healthy foods become even more enjoyable as your taste buds change and your body feels better as a result of the improved nutrition.

I know what some of you are thinking: "But, Diane, what if my sugar cravings *aren't* gone?" Hang in there! This program isn't magic. It takes time, and the amount of time it takes may vary for everyone. Some people need to continue to reinforce their new healthy habits for several more days, weeks, or even months after the 21DSD before they feel a *complete* shift in their cravings. For others, the shock to their system and the fact that the 21DSD forces them to find another way to feel good yanks them out of their cravings pattern quickly.

Give it time. You didn't develop these habits and cravings overnight, and they may not all disappear quickly. But I promise you this: they get so much better over time!

TODAY'S MEALS

Breakfast:
⅓ Pumpkin Spice Smoothie + 2 hard-boiled eggs

Lunch:
Leftover Grilled Pork Fall Salad

Dinner:
B3 Bowl (page 152)

Snack(s): 2 slices 21DSD Cinnamon Banana Bread + nut butter

> ❝ *Day 11! Feeling wonderful. Not hungry throughout the day. Feel less bloated. Sleeping really good. I absolutely love soda, but after a week or so on the program, the seltzer water + lime is seriously satisfying. So crisp and has a strong carbonation bite. I look forward to adopting this after the program.* ❞

— Jason S. (21DSD Community Member)

✎ NOTES ABOUT TODAY

I'm surprised that my cravings... _____

_____

_____

_____

One thing I find triggers my cravings is... _____

_____

_____

Ways that I can be present and observe why I feel a craving are... _____

_____

_____

notes _____

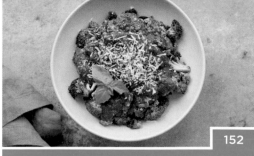

152

TODAY'S RECIPE
B3 Bowl

TODAY'S CHECKLIST

- [ ] **Check your stress.** Audit yourself to identify when you find yourself reaching for or craving sweets/carbs, if it's still happening. Is it when you're tired, angry, bored? Journal about this.

- [ ] **Prep** Broccoli, Ham & Cheese Frittata (page 136) for breakfast days 12 & 14.

- [ ] **Post to social media** using the hashtag #21DSD about your day 11 experience and share foods you find yourself craving that you never would have before!

SLEEP TIME & QUALITY

to bed last night _____

woke up today _____

- [ ] excellent
- [ ] fair
- [ ] good
- [ ] poor

EXERCISE

time _____

_____

type _____

MOOD & ENERGY

- [ ] excellent
- [ ] fair
- [ ] good
- [ ] poor

TODAY'S FRUIT

🍎 or 🍌 or 🍊

"I'm not feeling as strong in my workouts."

You may experience: Shakiness or weakness from going too low-carb; if you're an athlete or work out regularly, you may not be performing as well. Remember to add those activity carbs to your meals as needed.

Your best bet: Make sure that you're adding the appropriate carb sources to your post-workout meals—see pages 22 to 23 for more on building your plate and activity carbs.

The Dish from Diane

If your energy isn't quite what you had hoped it would be, jump back over to day 3 (page 48) and review what's happening with the balance on your plate. Don't try to be a hero here and restrict foods beyond what this program outlines.

I've seen it happen time and time again: someone bails out on the 21DSD because they are tired or hungry, but when asked about what they were eating and how active they were while on the program, it's so clear to me that adding good carbs would have made it so much easier for them! I want you to be successful, but I can't do it for you. You've got to take the reins here and eat plenty of those good foods—including carbs!

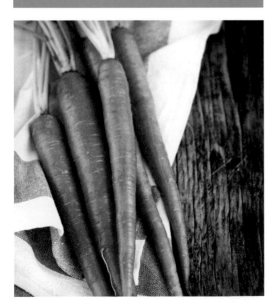

DAY 12

TODAY'S LESSON
Where's my energy?

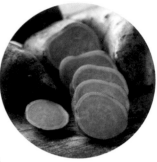

You're almost two weeks in right now, and you may be feeling awesome, or you may be wondering, "Where is all the energy other people keep talking about?! I just don't have it!" First, everyone's experience will vary from day to day and week to week on the 21DSD. That said, if your energy is plummeting, it's time to get real about how you're building your 21DSD plate.

I know that many people enter this program with the mindset that carbs are bad and you need to avoid them. I get it! This program is about helping you bust cravings not only for sugar but for carby, junky foods in general. So if you've been a bit hesitant to include more good carbs on your plate, it's not surprising.

But here's your wake-up call: your energy is likely tanking because your body wants more carbs! And that's okay! There are plenty of healthy good carbs for you to enjoy on the 21DSD. And I promise you this: eating more good carbs will not increase your cravings. In fact, when you eat good carbs, you'll actually satisfy those cravings in a healthy way! A sweet potato with some ghee and cinnamon is such a wonderful way to provide your body with good carbs, and I challenge you to sit quietly and really feel what your body is telling you after eating it. Perhaps your mind is trying to tell you that you want something more sugary, but I bet that your body feels better, calmer, and more at ease after that sweet potato.

Real food is so powerful when you ditch the junk and allow it to fuel you!

> "The future depends on what you do today."
>
> — Mahatma Gandhi

TODAY'S MEALS

Breakfast:
Broccoli, Ham & Cheese Frittata

Lunch:
Leftover BBQ Pulled Pork Tacos with Spicy Slaw

Dinner:
Creamy Mustard Chicken with Zoodles (page 174)

Snack(s): 2 slices 21DSD Cinnamon Banana Bread + nut butter

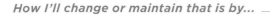

NOTES ABOUT TODAY

Recently my energy has been...

How I'll change or maintain that is by...

My favorite real-food carbs so far on the 21DSD have been...

notes

174

TODAY'S RECIPE
Creamy Mustard Chicken with Zoodles

TODAY'S CHECKLIST

☐ **Post to social media** using the hashtag #21DSD about your day 12 experience and favorite meals so far!

SLEEP TIME & QUALITY

to bed last night _____

woke up today _____

☐ excellent   ☐ fair

☐ good   ☐ poor

EXERCISE

time _____

type _____

MOOD & ENERGY

☐ excellent   ☐ fair

☐ good   ☐ poor

TODAY'S FRUIT

🍎 or 🍌 or 🍊

The Dish from Diane

As you approach your third week of this detox, you may be feeling like you've hit a stride and really have this whole thing down. You may even be feeling like this wouldn't be a bad way to eat in the long term. While I do want you to bring back some foods to your life post-21DSD (don't worry, it's all covered in your post-detox week!), I definitely don't want you to feel like eating 21DSD-style is the only way to be healthy. There are many ways to incorporate healthy foods that aren't 21DSD-friendly (like sweet fruits and berries) after your detox is completed, and we'll talk about that in your post-detox week.

Feeling like this hasn't been so easy? It's common at this point to feel like you've already done "enough," or like you've gotten what you needed from the detox. Stay the course! The next week is going to solidify a lot of the new healthy habits you're creating, and it'll challenge you to push outside your comfort zone when it comes to meal and snack creativity. I've got you covered with creative but easy meal ideas, so stick with me here! You *can* do this, and I've got your back!

DAY 13

TODAY'S LESSON

Sugar and inflammation

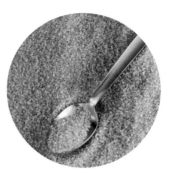

Have you noticed that some aches and pains, or maybe some skin irritation or acne you used to struggle with, have started calming down? Wondering why stripping sugar from your diet is having this great effect? It's all about lowering inflammation in your body.

Inflammation is the body's response to a problem. When your body thinks there's a constant problem, it lives in a chronic state of inflammation. This steady, low-level inflammatory state underlies all chronic disease and suppressed immunity. Essentially, it's at the root of just about every disease or dis-ease state (big or small) imaginable.

Sugar consumption plays a role in chronic inflammation in two main ways:

1. Depleted nutrient stores from overconsumption of bad carbs (see page 62 for more on how bad carbs deplete your nutrients) lead to a chronic state of stress in the body, and that means inflammation.

2. Chronically high and/or low blood sugar—that blood sugar roller coaster that comes from consistently ingesting too many bad carbs—creates a stress state for the body, and again, that means inflammation.

Now that you've removed sugar and poor-quality carbs from your diet, your systemic inflammation is dropping, and you may be seeing the results in myriad ways: better skin, improved digestion, fewer symptoms from chronic conditions, and more. This is one of the many ways that diet impacts our health in more ways than we imagine!

"**Every accomplishment begins with a decision to try.**"

— Edward T. Kelly

TODAY'S MEALS

Breakfast:
Leftover Breakfast Salad

Lunch:
Leftover Creamy Mustard Chicken with Zoodles

Dinner:
Leftover B3 Bowl

Snack(s): Smoky Toasted Nut Mix or jerky

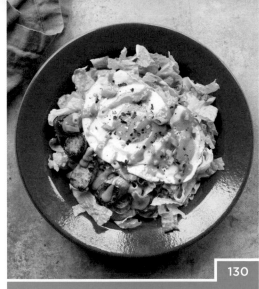

130

TODAY'S RECIPE
Breakfast Salad

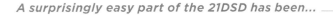

✎ NOTES ABOUT TODAY

Something I will no longer sweeten as much is...

A surprisingly easy part of the 21DSD has been...

One thing I want to continue to do better is...

notes

TODAY'S CHECKLIST

☐ **Post to social media** using the hashtag #21DSD about your day 13 experience and share an ache or pain that's cleared up since starting the program!

SLEEP TIME & QUALITY

to bed last night _____

woke up today_____

☐ excellent   ☐ fair

☐ good   ☐ poor

EXERCISE

time _____

type _____

MOOD & ENERGY

☐ excellent   ☐ fair

☐ good   ☐ poor

TODAY'S FRUIT

🍎 or 🍌 or 🍊

WHAT TO EXPECT

"I'm sleeping like a baby—is this for real?"

You may experience: Not only falling asleep faster but also sleeping better through the night and waking up feeling more well rested.

Your best bet: Continue to cultivate good sleep habits (getting to bed and waking up at consistent times daily; sleeping in a dark, cool room; and following a nightly routine) to ensure that you get enough sleep through the rest of the detox and beyond.

The Dish from Diane

As much as I encourage you to consume foods rich in nutrients that support melatonin production, I strongly recommend *against* using a melatonin supplement to help you sleep unless you're advised to do so by a medical professional. Melatonin is a hormone, and the goal should be to support your body in producing it naturally. Taking it in a supplement form may cause a variety of problems, including but not limited to the following: disrupted sleep patterns, vivid dreams, grogginess, headaches, daytime sleepiness, short-term feelings of depression, dizziness, stomach cramps, and irritability. Let your nutrition support your body naturally!

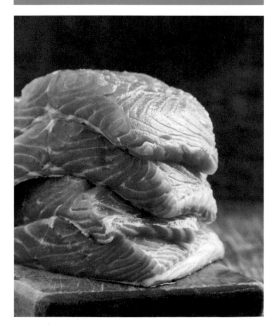

DAY 14

TODAY'S LESSON
I'm sleeping better, but why?

Getting off the blood sugar roller coaster has positive benefits that reach far beyond busting sugar cravings. Some of the biggest benefits: more-stable energy throughout the day, better mental sharpness, and improved sleep!

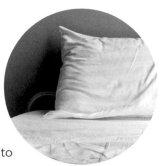

Why? Well, when your blood sugar isn't alternately spiking and crashing throughout the day, your body's stress response is lowered, which leads to an easier time falling asleep and more restful sleep. Furthermore, when you have more energy throughout the day, you can *expend* more energy, which also leads to more restful sleep.

Another big reason why your sleep could be improving on the 21DSD: nutrition! You're now getting more zinc, vitamin B6, and the amino acid tryptophan, all of which help your body make melatonin, the hormone responsible for regulating our sleep and wake cycle—meaning your body needs healthy levels of them in order to support healthy sleep!

Which foods are we talking about here?

21DSD foods rich in zinc	21DSD foods rich in vitamin B6
beef	beef
cashews	chicken
lamb	plantains and bananas
pumpkin seeds	potatoes
sesame seeds and tahini	salmon
shrimp	spinach
turkey	sweet potatoes
	sunflower seeds
	tuna
	turkey

If sleep is an area you'd like to focus on during (or after) your 21DSD, be sure you're eating plenty of these foods!

TODAY'S MEALS

Breakfast:	Lunch:	Dinner:
Leftover Broccoli, Ham & Cheese Frittata	Deli Tuna Sliders (page 178)	Diane's Simple Roast Chicken (170) + Pesto Roasted Carrots (198) + Ranch Roasted Potatoes (206)

Snack(s): 2 slices 21DSD Cinnamon Banana Bread + nut butter

> **"** *Day 13 and the sleep I am getting is unbelievable. The past 2 mornings I have woken in the morning feeling fantastic. #detoxsleeprocks* **"**
>
> — Jessica M. (21DSD Community Member)

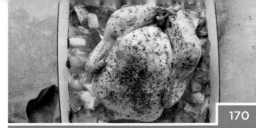

170

TODAY'S RECIPE
Diane's Simple Roast Chicken

TODAY'S CHECKLIST

- [ ] **Prep** Apple Pie Smoothie (page 144) and hard-boil 6 eggs for breakfast days 15, 18 & 20.
- [ ] **Prep** Two-Bite Chocolate Cream Pies (page 218) and Smoky Toasted Nut Mix (page 212) for snacks.
- [ ] **Prep** sauces and condiments per the meal plan, page 119.
- [ ] **Post to social media** using the hashtag #21DSD about your day 14 experience and share any positive changes you've experienced with your sleep.

NOTES ABOUT TODAY

Lately my sleep has been... _____

_____

_____

_____

How I'll change or maintain that is by... _____

_____

_____

_____

My favorite way to unwind for a good night's sleep is... _____

_____

_____

_____

notes _____

_____

SLEEP TIME & QUALITY

to bed last night _____

woke up today _____

- [ ] excellent
- [ ] fair
- [ ] good
- [ ] poor

EXERCISE

time _____

_____

type _____

MOOD & ENERGY

- [ ] excellent
- [ ] fair
- [ ] good
- [ ] poor

TODAY'S FRUIT

🍎 or 🍌 or 🍊

"Not. Another. Green. Apple."

You may experience: Boredom with food choices and longing for foods that you have eliminated. (There's a lot of variety in the meal plan, so if you're following that, maybe you're not experiencing this at all.) Perhaps at first you were pretty excited about the fact that you could have some fruit on the 21DSD. By now, however, your giddiness over a green apple or an underripe banana or grapefruit may have faded.

Your best bet: Expand the foods you eat by one or two new proteins or cuts, two new vegetables, and a new spice blend or two. You won't know what new flavors you love until you try them!

The Dish from Diane

As you head into this last week, I don't want you thinking about how the detox is a black-and-white period of time where you ate a certain way, and life after your detox will be totally different. I want you to think about all the grey areas where you can find yourself eating the real, whole, nutrient-dense foods you've come to love on the program as part of your routine. The real benefits from this program are the lessons you learn, not simply the three weeks of time while you follow it. In order to reap the same amazing benefits that thousands of other participants have over the years, you need to take responsibility here. The choices you make most of the time matter more than the ones you make for a short amount of time. In other words, this detox can change your life, but only if you let it!

"**Don't give up when you still have something to give. Nothing is really over until the moment you stop trying.**"

— Brian Dyson

DAY 15

TODAY'S LESSON
Reigniting your motivation

This is it, your last week on the 21DSD. The mixed emotions that come with this week can be both liberating and challenging at the same time. On the one hand, you're hitting a major stride with your preparation, building meals, and recognizing your own personal stressors and sugar/carb-eating triggers. On the other hand, you may be doubting the value of yet another full week of this program:

Maybe all I need are two weeks?

I think I have this thing down, maybe the last week is pointless?

I've made it far enough, haven't I?

These are all potential negative mindsets that you may have as you enter into this final week. And I'm here to shut that down right now!

First and foremost, I want you to be so proud that you've gotten through the first two weeks! That is huge. It really is. But those two weeks are not the full program, and I can't make any promises about how much better you'll feel or whether you'll get the full benefits of the program if you cut it 33 percent short. I need you to hang in there and finish out this last week strong!

Channel your strength into simplifying everything you've been doing to keep moving forward on this detox. For instance, take note of when you can save leftovers to use in another recipe, or when you see a 21DSD-friendly snack that you can stash in your purse or desk drawer at the office. Work the lessons you're learning into your daily life and find ways to make small changes in your thought process about how you approach meals throughout the day.

Finishing the 21DSD isn't about just going back to how you ate before the detox! It's about incorporating the healthy lessons you've learned into your life beyond the 21DSD. Sure, you'll eat more things post-detox than you do now, but you won't throw away what you've learned about healthy eating or what feels good for your body. So start paying close attention now to what you'll plan to continue doing once the three weeks end. Don't worry, I'm going to guide you through your post-detox week to help you make that shift, but right now, just get the wheels turning and trust that you *can* and *will* keep a lot of these healthy habits going!

TODAY'S MEALS

Breakfast:
⅓ Apple Pie Smoothie + 2 hard-boiled eggs

Lunch:
Buddha bowl with leftover roast chicken, pesto, carrots & potatoes

Dinner:
Grilled steak (see page 120) + Roasted Eggplant Steaks with Tahini Sauce (page 208)

Snack(s): Smoky Toasted Nut Mix or jerky

> ❝ *I'm on day 15 and today I feel like I hit a wall. I'm exhausted and starving tonight. Thankfully I have bacon already cooked and an easy dinner that is compliant. Before this I would have eaten junk or fast food, but thankfully I've learned and prepped enough to keep it healthy tonight.* ❞
>
> – Jacquelyn H. (21DSD Community Member)

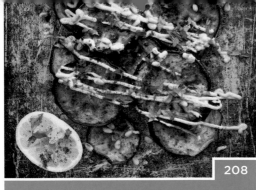

208

TODAY'S RECIPE
Roasted Eggplant Steaks + Tahini Sauce

TODAY'S CHECKLIST

- [ ] **Prep** Roasted Butternut Squash (page 202) for lunch days 17 & 19.

- [ ] **Prep** Mushroom, Pesto & Goat Cheese Frittata (page 134) for breakfast day 16, using mushrooms from day 12.

- [ ] **Post to social media** using the hashtag #21DSD about your day 15 experience and share one way you will incorporate your new healthy habits into your life after the 21DSD.

✎ NOTES ABOUT TODAY

Something that almost got me off-track but didn't was...

_____
_____
_____

I'm feeling really proud that... _____
_____
_____
_____

I know that a healthy habit I'll continue after the 21DSD is...
_____
_____
_____

notes _____
_____

SLEEP TIME & QUALITY

to bed last night _____
woke up today _____

- [ ] excellent
- [ ] good
- [ ] fair
- [ ] poor

EXERCISE

time _____

type _____

MOOD & ENERGY

- [ ] excellent
- [ ] good
- [ ] fair
- [ ] poor

TODAY'S FRUIT

🍎 or 🍌 or 🍊

"I know this isn't a weight-loss plan, but I was secretly hoping that I would lose some weight!"

You may experience: Some movement on the scale or (even better) extra room in your clothes. But you may not see this, even if you're getting healthier.

Your best bet: Step away from the scale. It's best not to get on the scale except once before and once after your 21DSD—otherwise, you'll drive yourself crazy watching those numbers. Instead, review the many reasons why you decided to begin this detox in the first place and focus on the amazing changes that have happened in your body and your life so far.

The Dish from Diane

Throw away your scale. I'm serious. I haven't owned a bathroom scale in probably more than ten years, and I'll tell you what, I'm happier for it.

Yes, the scale does provide *some* information: it tells you about the Earth's gravitational pull on your body. But you can get better-quality information about your health in more ways than we can count. How do your clothes fit? How is your energy? Your performance in the gym. Your moods. Your skin. Your more positive mental attitude overall. Need I go on? These are all better ways to evaluate your health than weighing yourself.

If you're concerned about overall weight loss, trust how your clothes fit, photos you take along the way to track progress, and basic body measurements (the kind you use to determine your clothing size) rather than the scale. If you are exercising, you're likely building muscle and losing fat, and that won't reflect in the way you're hoping it will on the scale. Don't forget that body fat weighs less than muscle mass—you could weigh less than someone of similar stature and still have more body fat.

DAY 16

TODAY'S LESSON
Portion size tips

While all of the recipes in this book were created with a certain portion size in mind, that doesn't mean that those portions are necessarily the right ones for you! You probably won't find you want less food, but you may find that you need more of certain things. There truly is no one prescription or formula for portion size, so here's how to figure out what's right for you.

Step 1: Know your starting point.

It's really hard to improve your satiety after meals—and figure out if more food or less food would be sufficient for you—if you don't know where you're starting. If you feel like you're not full for long enough after meals, or if you serve yourself meals over and over again that you can't finish, start by measuring out the portion of each dish with a food scale, measuring cups, and/or measuring spoons. But please don't let this make you crazy or obsessive about portions—it's simply information.

Measure your portions for several days so you get a good overall sense of how much you are eating and what your portion sizes look like. Realistically, you won't be around these measuring tools all the time, so you'll want to learn how to eyeball amounts—this week of measuring should help with that!

Pay close attention to how much you are eating and how you feel afterward. You may notice that you need closer to six ounces of meat when you were only eating four ounces at a time. Focus on feeling full and satisfied. You're measuring for information, not deprivation!

Step 2: Test, test, test.

Now you need to test how you feel with different portions. For each meal, track:

- which foods you ate
- how much you ate of each food
- when you ate
- how you felt before and after eating

Be sure to write down how long the meal kept you full, when (and if) you got "hangry," and how long after that meal you needed to eat again. All this varies for each and every person, and it may change depending on the type of exercise you do on a particular day, your overall lifestyle, or even the amount of stress you have.

It's important to learn how to test and adjust your portions because life factors constantly change…which leads to step 3.

Step 3: Balance your plate, then balance it again.

Pay attention to how your body responds when you add more of one type of food to your plate. If it's not the result you want, then rebalance your plate, being mindful of your portions, and try to shift something different the next time you change it. Perhaps you need to add more protein to feel your best, or perhaps more fat. You may find you need to add a little more of both protein and fat, or just one or the other. The satiety you'll feel as a result of these shifts varies from person to person, so rebalancing your plate for your own appetite needs is key. Also note if your activity level has changed—that will change how you will balance your plate (most likely, if you're moving more, you'll need more protein and healthy carbs).

Many people have told me that when they added more carbs to their plate, they gained weight. Often this happens because you're adding calories (in the form of healthy carbs) to your plate without readjusting what was on your plate already. If you want to add healthy carbs without increasing your overall calorie intake, then you'll need to adjust your intake of protein (somewhat) and fats (mostly) to avoid overeating.

TODAY'S MEALS

Breakfast:	Lunch:	Dinner:
Mushroom, Pesto & Goat Cheese Frittata + *leftover* Ranch Roasted Potatoes	*Leftover* Deli Tuna Sliders	Mediterranean Meatball Bowl (page 180)

Snack(s): Two-Bite Chocolate Cream Pies

✎ NOTES ABOUT TODAY

One food type I will continue to eat more of is... _____

_____

_____

Something I've realized I may overdo easily is... _____

_____

_____

A win I've had recently is... _____

_____

_____

notes _____

_____

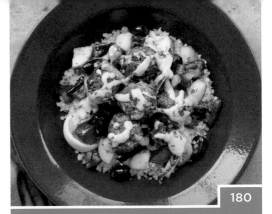

180

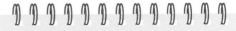

TODAY'S CHECKLIST

☐ **Throw away your scale.** Yes, really.

☐ **Prep** 1 head roasted garlic for dinner day 18.

☐ **Prep** chicken thighs for lunch days 17 & 19.

☐ **Post to social media** using the hashtag #21DSD about your day 16 experience and a photo of your scale in the trash can.

SLEEP TIME & QUALITY

to bed last night _____

woke up today _____

☐ excellent   ☐ fair

☐ good   ☐ poor

EXERCISE

time _____

_____

type _____

_____

MOOD & ENERGY

☐ excellent   ☐ fair

☐ good   ☐ poor

TODAY'S FRUIT

🍎 or 🍌 or 🍊

You may experience: Feelings of impatience for the end of the detox. Day 17 is almost like "hump day" on the 21DSD.

Your best bet: Keep checking in with friends who are on the detox with you and with supporters you've met online. Think of a non-food reward that you'll "win" at the end of the twenty-one days—buy that cookbook you've had your eye on, get a manicure, treat yourself to a day at a museum, go to a play or concert, buy tickets to a sporting event, or outfit your kitchen with some new tools.

The Dish from Diane

This one may hit you *hard*. At a signing event for *The 21-Day Sugar Detox* in Texas several years ago, a woman asked, "What can I snack on at work?" Now, to the untrained ear, this question is very straightforward. She wanted to know what to eat when hunger hit during business hours while on the 21DSD, right? Wrong.

My response shocked everyone in the room, including the woman asking the question. Rather than provide simple ideas like some roasted almonds and an apple, jerky and carrot sticks, or nut butter and a green-tipped banana (all great 21DSD snack ideas, by the way), I asked her if she was truly hungry for a snack or if she might be bored at work, leading her to get up and look for a snack around 2 or 3 p.m. every day. To the surprise of the room, she replied, "Actually, I think I'm bored."

Not long after that event, she emailed me to tell me she had quit her job and was happily pursuing more meaningful and interesting work, and that she was so thankful for the way that I responded to her seemingly simple question about snacking! I challenge you to discover whether or not you're truly hungry for a snack while at work, or if you're simply bored or restless with what you're doing. If it's the latter, a snack is never going to solve that "hunger."

DAY 17

TODAY'S LESSON
To snack or not to snack?

While there are snack options in the daily meal plan, it's not something that's set up as a "need to eat." You may find on your 21DSD that you truly need a snack every day, or you may find that once you balance your plate differently (see day 16) you no longer need snacks.

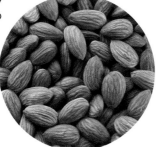

Here are a few things to keep in mind when deciding whether or not to snack, as well as some thoughts on what to snack on if you do need an extra nibble between meals:

1. **Consider whether you're truly hungry or simply bored, restless, or tired.** If you aren't truly hungry, then the snack isn't going to help. Take a few moments to assess how you're feeling and what is at the root of that feeling. If you feel that you are truly hungry, then eat something. This program isn't about starvation or deprivation!

2. **Pay attention to when you get hungry for a snack.** If it's consistently at the same time each day, could you have eaten more at the previous meal to avoid getting hungry? For example, if you eat breakfast at 8 a.m. and find that you're hungry at 10 or 11 a.m., maybe an extra egg or sausage can help you stave off hunger until lunch. Or if you're hungry after you ate a green salad for lunch and skimped on the protein and healthy fats, then consider larger portions next time. The time of day you feel like a snack may also point to whether or not you're truly hungry: if you consistently feel hungry at 3 p.m. when you're in a long stretch at work, maybe it's not that you didn't eat enough at lunch—maybe you're bored.

Your meals should sustain you for at least three hours, if not much longer. This may sound contrary to what many of us were told for years, but if you're eating well-balanced meals with healthy fats, it's a good benchmark. You also want to get hungry for your next meal, but not "hangry." (Review the difference on page 5.) If you need more food, have more food, but I'd encourage you not to plan to eat snacks but rather to make your meals a bit larger, so they satiate you for longer. This gives your body time between meals to appropriately digest and absorb nutrients and helps regulate blood sugar and appetite.

3. **Be prepared.** Sound familiar? If you've got healthy 21DSD-friendly snacks on hand, like homemade trail mix; some jerky that's free of sugar, gluten, and soy; plain roasted nuts; some cheese (Levels 1 and 2 only); or an avocado, you'll be ready if hunger strikes! Being prepared is at least 90 percent of being able to avoid temptation to go off the rails. Simply having the right foods on hand and ready to go means your snacks will be healthy and balanced.

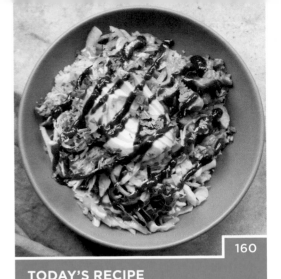

160

TODAY'S RECIPE
BBQ Pulled Pork Buddha Bowl

TODAY'S MEALS

Breakfast:	Lunch:	Dinner:
Leftover Mushroom, Pesto & Goat Cheese Frittata + *leftover* Ranch Roasted Potatoes	BBQ Chicken Salad (page 156)	BBQ Pulled Pork Buddha Bowl (page 160)

Snack(s): Two-Bite Chocolate Cream Pies

✎ NOTES ABOUT TODAY

A favorite snack of mine on the 21DSD has been... _____

_____

_____

_____

I noticed that I reach for a snack when I'm not necessarily hungry but... _____

_____

_____

_____

One way I can tell if I'm truly hungry or not is... _____

_____

_____

_____

notes _____

TODAY'S CHECKLIST

☐ **Post to social media** using the hashtag #21DSD about your day 17 experience and share your own discoveries about snack-seeking and any boredom-based hunger moments.

SLEEP TIME & QUALITY

to bed last night _____

woke up today _____

☐ excellent ☐ fair

☐ good ☐ poor

EXERCISE

time _____

_____

type _____

MOOD & ENERGY

☐ excellent ☐ fair

☐ good ☐ poor

TODAY'S FRUIT

🍎 or 🍌 or 🍊

"I really am in the home stretch now, but what am I going to do after this?"

You may experience: Some anxiety about what you'll do after the twenty-one days are up—this is normal.

Your best bet: Stay the course, and peek ahead to preview the post-detox week if it'll help you feel like you know what to expect. Think about whole, healthy foods that you want to introduce back to your plate first, such as sweeter fruits.

The Dish from Diane

Today's lesson is all about knowing yourself better so that you can make better choices as you transition to life after the detox. The process isn't always a linear one. You may start out thinking that you can moderate certain foods, only to discover that you're best off avoiding them completely. Or you may think that banning certain foods completely will help you and find that it doesn't. What works best isn't the same for everyone, and I'd argue that it's also not the same for each person with different foods.

For example, you may find that you have no problem strictly abstaining from gluten-containing foods in the future. Maybe it seems like no big deal, because you feel better without gluten and gluten-free options are easy to find. But at the same time, you may find that if you try to abstain from cheese and other dairy foods, you feel overly drawn to them. So, whether you abstain from or moderate certain foods may vary from food to food—and that's okay. Being aware of yourself and what works best for you is the goal here, and I want for you to feel released from the constant turmoil around food that makes you question yourself. You are the boss of yourself and your choices—move forward from here confident in that fact!

DAY 18

TODAY'S LESSON
Thinking about life after the 21DSD

You've got four whole days left on the program. And don't even think about cutting this short—you are worth finishing this thing you started! You've made it THIS. FAR. Stopping short at this point would be a total bummer. Don't let yourself down by throwing in the towel now.

The finish line is fully in sight, and your momentum towards it may either be super strong ("I HAVE SO GOT THIS!"), or it may slightly be waning ("Do I *really* need to finish these next several days?"). So, here's what to do: begin thinking about—and planning—your post-detox life!

The daily entries for the post-detox week (pages 90 to 103) have some suggestions for thoughtful tweaks to your nutrition and how to add foods back to your plate, so you're covered there. But what you can do now is to wrap your head around the idea that after the 21DSD, you're not going to go on a gluten-and-sugar bender. I've seen it far too many times—folks want to just "eat all the food" again. I get it. This program is not easy!

But when you thoughtfully and carefully bring foods back to your plate, you allow yourself space for awareness and insight, a moment to think about how what you eat affects how you feel. From there, you can make conscious decisions about what you'll eat going forward. The goal isn't to eat 21DSD-style for life! I want you to take these three weeks and learn from them, then apply what works for you going forward.

Take stock of how you handled the not-sweet treats throughout the program. Did you find that including them helped you stay on track more easily? Or did they distract you or make you feel like you couldn't have just the portion outlined for you? Have you found over the years that you do better completely avoiding something that you don't respond well to (whether with cravings, allergies, or emotional eating), or do you feel that when you tell yourself you can't have *any,* you feel even more drawn to those foods?

If you find that eating a little bit of a treat pushes you into a downward spiral that doesn't feel good, then abstaining from certain foods is a better approach for you.

On the flip side, if you find that by eating a little bit of something sweet rather than telling yourself you can't have a single bite, you feel more balanced, sane, and calm around those foods, then for you, the concept of moderation is a good one.

Learning whether you do better by abstaining from or moderating foods that can be triggers for you is a worthwhile endeavor. This way of knowing yourself better will allow you to feel less controlled by food and calmer around foods that you know can be triggers for you.

READ UP!

I highly recommend the book Better Than Before, *by Gretchen Rubin, to help you figure out whether you do better abstaining from or moderating certain foods.*

TODAY'S MEALS

Breakfast:	Lunch:	Dinner:
⅓ Apple Pie Smoothie + 2 hard-boiled eggs	*Leftover* Mediterranean Meatball Bowl	Sausage & Spinach "Polenta" Bowl (page 186)

Snack(s): Smoky Toasted Nut Mix or jerky

✎ NOTES ABOUT TODAY

For me, moderation works/doesn't work because... _____

_____

_____

_____

I've discovered that I'm better than I thought at... _____

_____

_____

_____

For the last few days of my 21DSD, I'm going to focus on...

_____

_____

_____

notes _____

_____

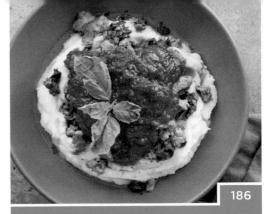

186

TODAY'S RECIPE
Sausage & Spinach "Polenta" Bowl

TODAY'S CHECKLIST

- [ ] **Prep** Sausage, Spinach & Peppers Frittata (page 138) for breakfast day 19 & lunch day 20.

- [ ] **Post to social media** using the hashtag #21DSD about day 18 and share your personal discoveries about whether you do better abstaining or moderating.

SLEEP TIME & QUALITY

to bed last night _____

woke up today _____

- [ ] excellent
- [ ] good
- [ ] fair
- [ ] poor

EXERCISE

time _____

_____

type _____

_____

MOOD & ENERGY

- [ ] excellent
- [ ] good
- [ ] fair
- [ ] poor

TODAY'S FRUIT

🍎 or 🍌 or 🍊

"This is close enough to 21 days, right? A little bit of [insert food you've been missing here] won't hurt, will it?"

You may experience: A strong urge to throw in the towel or call it "good enough."

Your best bet: Keep your eyes on the prize. Remember that this detox is not just about getting sugar out of your life for three weeks; it's also about changing your mindset toward food and your habits. When you make it through just three more days, the feeling of accomplishment will be awesome!

The Dish from Diane

As you finish out this program, remember that post-21DSD, you don't need to put pressure on yourself to eat this way for forever—that can feel overwhelming. Don't freak yourself out or worry that you'll fall off the rails. Rather than challenge yourself to "stick to it," approach your upcoming weeks and days just as you've approached your weeks and days on the program. Plan and prep meals and snacks for the week so you don't leave too much of your nutrition to chance, and include some healthy, whole foods that weren't included before, like fruits. You already know that if you don't have any healthy snacks in your purse or desk, the options you'll find won't be the best for you. And you knew this before the 21DSD.

Make your choices moment to moment, checking in with yourself as you go and not automatically saying yes to treats you don't truly want simply because you're not on the 21DSD anymore. Set yourself up for success by continuing to think ahead about your meals after the detox. You know you still need to eat every single day, so move ahead with that knowledge, and keep it as healthy as you can and want to!

DAY 19

TODAY'S LESSON
Don't get stuck in a goal-setting trap

We've talked at length about finding your "why" as well as what it takes to stick to this program you've committed to. So what happens when you reach the goal you've set by completing this program? How do you move ahead *mentally* once you've reached the goal of completing the 21-Day Sugar Detox?

This is why planning for sustainability and making your goal *learning,* rather than fixating on the endpoint, is effective. You've made a lot of changes to your everyday habits and ways of eating on the 21DSD. Take a moment now to reflect on that, and take in everything you can from this experience. Remember all the situations you've faced—lunch meetings, eating out with friends, weeknight meals—and how the choices you made were very different from those you would have made if you had not been on the program. What was your thought process in those situations? Were there moments when you realized that you truly didn't need to add sweetener to something, or when you were happy to opt for your included fruit rather than cake that might leave you feeling "off"?

All of those thought processes are reasonable and valid, and worth exploring. When you realize that you have the free will to choose to eat whatever you want, whenever you want, you then realize that you also have the freedom to say no to foods that you don't truly want because you'd rather feel great overall—even if you have a moment of wanting those foods.

So far I've been cheering you on and keeping you focused on following and finishing the 21DSD, and that's because keeping focus in the moment is critical. But now, rather than looking at your progress through these three weeks as simply powering through the program and then returning to your old ways, it's time to transition to a goal of finding your own new way of eating that works well for you.

TODAY'S MEALS

Breakfast:
Sausage, Spinach & Peppers Frittata

Lunch:
Leftover BBQ Chicken Salad

Dinner:
Leftover BBQ Pulled Pork Buddha Bowl

Snack(s): Two-Bite Chocolate Cream Pies

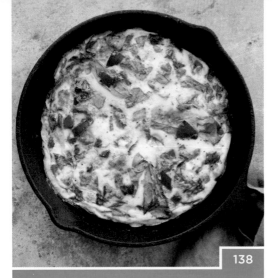

138

TODAY'S RECIPE
Sausage, Spinach & Peppers Frittata

> *Day 19 and I was soooooooo tempted to buy wine tonight. I didn't. Opened up my book and looked at what to expect on day 19. Sure enough, it said you may experience a strong urge to cheat or call it good enough at 19 days. The urge was strong, but I was stronger.*

— Natalie C. (21DSD Community Member)

TODAY'S CHECKLIST

☐ **Post to social media** using the hashtag #21DSD about your day 19 experience and share some new ways you're thinking about healthy foods and sweets.

NOTES ABOUT TODAY

Rather than the end of this program, I see day 21 as the beginning of...

_____
_____
_____

Some healthy foods I'm excited to enjoy when the detox ends are...

_____
_____
_____

One stressor that I've learned causes me to reach for sugar is...

_____
_____
_____

notes _____
_____

SLEEP TIME & QUALITY

to bed last night _____

woke up today _____

☐ excellent   ☐ fair

☐ good   ☐ poor

EXERCISE

time _____
_____

type _____
_____

MOOD & ENERGY

☐ excellent   ☐ fair

☐ good   ☐ poor

TODAY'S FRUIT

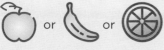 or 🍌 or ⊗

"On day 22, I'm going to go crazy and eat everything I want!"

You may experience: A strong desire to plan an all-out carb-fest.

Your best bet: Focus on these last two days and finish up strong! Worry about day 22 when it comes, not today!

The Dish from Diane

You may feel so amazing right now that you never want to eat sugar again! And while that's a truly noble thought and perhaps a worthwhile effort as well, I don't think it's realistic. Yes, you read that correctly. The creator of the 21-Day Sugar Detox doesn't think it's realistic to never eat a bite of sugar again.

Here's the thing: I don't want a perfectionist mindset to get you all caught up! There is a healthy way to enjoy sweet foods (and treats!) once you've figured out how you personally feel—mentally, emotionally, and physically—when you eat them. For weeks, months, even years beyond the 21DSD, you'll be faced with the decision of whether to eat a treat or not. Each time you decide to eat it, you'll see how you feel after you eat it. Are you able to enjoy a treat and move on? Are you riddled with guilt or shame? Do you physically feel ill?

No one is going to be sitting on your shoulder, waving a finger and saying "You shouldn't eat that" for the rest of your life. In fact, I don't want to encourage your own inner dialogue to be even close to that. When you release the power that food has over your emotions and realize that you can make a choice to enjoy a treat and then move on and return to your regular, everyday food, having a treat will no longer be the start of a downward spiral it may have once been.

DAY 20

TODAY'S LESSON
How to reintroduce foods after your 21DSD

Ultimately, it's up to you to choose what foods you'll add back into your regularly scheduled food programming, and how often, but before you bury yourself in a pile of grain-free baked goods or a bottle of wine, consider the following:

- How do you feel now that you've changed your food?

- How do you think you'll feel if you eat a particular food that you estimate is less than healthy for you?

- If you think you'll feel less than optimal, how long will that feeling last? More than a couple of hours? More than a day? More than a week?

- Will a particular food disrupt blood sugar regulation or digestive function? Mental clarity? The sense of accomplishment you have from not eating it for the past three weeks?

- Have the time and energy you've put into avoiding a particular food added more stress to your life than eliminating it alleviated symptoms of ill health?

When you consider these questions, you'll become a lot more mindful of your food choices, rather than defaulting to certain foods simply out of habit or convenience.

Adding back sugars and starches

To safely and slowly add some naturally occurring sugars (like fruit) and starches back into your diet, take care to consider the portions and timing of these foods. Avoid eating fruits alone if you have had problems with blood sugar regulation and cravings. Eat small portions of berries or half a piece of fruit if you're not a very active person, or larger portions if you are more active.

If you simply want to avoid cravings and you feel okay (perhaps even better?) when you resume eating some starchy foods, then you can enjoy root vegetables, tubers like sweet potatoes, and squash more frequently.

Reintroducing specific foods

- **Fruit:** Whole, fresh fruit can certainly have a regularly appearing role in your diet, but it's important to find a balance and not overdo it.

- **Grass-fed dairy (if you were on Level 3):** Missing your yogurt? Try adding it back in and see how you do. I recommend buying only grass-fed forms of dairy to consume in your home, but you may find you can enjoy goat cheese in an omelet while dining out with no ill effects. Or not. See how it goes for you.

- **Dark chocolate:** I'm talking 80 to 85 percent cacao or more—it's lower in sugar and a good source of antioxidants. Most folks don't tend to overindulge in too much when it's super dark. Look for an organic chocolate, preferably soy-free.

- **Gluten-free grains or legumes:** If you want to test how you do with these, white rice, quinoa, and black beans are all good choices to add in and track.

- **A glass of wine:** I'm not saying you should drink daily after your detox, but it's often a good idea to find out how you feel after consuming wine again if you previously drank. Perhaps it won't trigger cravings for you or you won't have any hangover effects. If that's the case, a glass once or twice a week may work well for you.

I'll walk you through some of these reintroductions in your post-detox week!

TODAY'S MEALS

Breakfast:	Lunch:	Dinner:
⅓ Apple Pie Smoothie + 2 hard-boiled eggs	*Leftover* Sausage, Spinach & Peppers Frittata + green salad	Super Garlic Meatballs with Fried Rice (page 184)

Snack(s): Smoky Toasted Nut Mix or jerky

✎ NOTES ABOUT TODAY

The food I plan to reintroduce first after the detox is... _____

_____

_____

One thing I'll especially look out for upon reintroducing food is...

_____

_____

Knowing tomorrow is the last official day of this program feels...

_____

_____

notes _____

_____

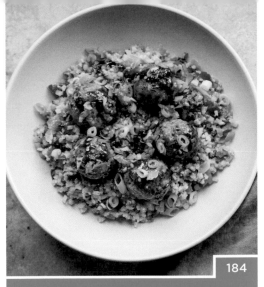
184

TODAY'S CHECKLIST

- [ ] **Post to social media** using the hashtag #21DSD about your day 20 experience and share a non-food treat you're going to enjoy on day 22.

SLEEP TIME & QUALITY

to bed last night _____

woke up today _____

- [ ] excellent
- [ ] fair
- [ ] good
- [ ] poor

EXERCISE

time _____

_____

type _____

MOOD & ENERGY

- [ ] excellent
- [ ] fair
- [ ] good
- [ ] poor

TODAY'S FRUIT

🍎 or 🍌 or 🍊

"This is it!"

You may experience: Relief, pride, excitement, and sheer joy that you made it to day 21!

Your best bet: Finish this day out strong. Get your head on straight about what tomorrow will bring, and hang with me here for your post-detox week of support and guidance—I'm not leaving you hanging!

The Dish from Diane

YOU DID IT! I'm proud of you. I hope you're proud of you, too. This program is challenging, to say the least. It's rare that anyone gets through the three weeks without a few bumps or struggles, and I want you to know that it's a *big* deal to say you've completed all twenty-one days. My next hope for you is that you can see exactly what kinds of other hard things you're capable of doing now that this is behind you. If you can do *this,* what else can you do that you didn't think you could? I can't wait to hear from you about all of those things, and I hope you'll stay connected with me via social media channels or through the website at 21daysugardetox. com.

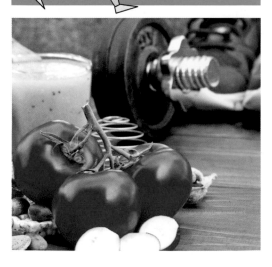

DAY 21

TODAY'S LESSON

Break free from someone else's plan, program, or rules

What the 21-Day Sugar Detox program does is release you from the chains that sugar and carbs may have had on you before you began. Remember that feeling you used to get after every meal where you couldn't help wanting or even needing something sweet to eat? Or the 3 p.m. afternoon sugar crash when your coworker would tempt you with the candy bowl? Do they feel like a distant memory? Good! While these cravings have subsided during this program, the ability to make healthier choices on autopilot have strengthened.

This program has worked to detox your body and your life in three distinct ways:

- **Your blood sugar and energy levels:** Now your body is more naturally efficient at burning fat for fuel and supporting your liver, which improves your metabolism and ability to regulate your blood sugar levels. This will impact your life in more areas than you can even imagine: sleep, gym, immune system, and more!

- **Taste buds:** Your palate's ability to adapt is truly astounding. Before, your palate was on overdrive from the sugar added to either sweeten foods or serve as a preservative for shelf-stable items, which left you with an increased tolerance for sweetness day after day. Since you've removed these sweeteners and overly sweet foods, you can appreciate how sweet whole, natural foods like beets and carrots can be.

- **Habits:** First and foremost, you could not have completed these last three full weeks of the 21-Day Sugar Detox without creating at least one new habit! A habit is a task you no longer have to think or stress about; the decisions have become automatic. When making good food choices is a habit, it's true freedom— and exactly why you'll stay on the right track tomorrow, and the day after, and the day after!

Now that you have a handle on what happens in your own body when you eat only 21DSD-friendly foods, you've got a great sense of what works for you and what doesn't! In the following week, you'll learn even more about how foods you reintroduce impact your body, and with that knowledge, combined with what you've learned from the last three weeks, you'll be equipped to choose your own way of eating that nourishes you in a healthy way.

TODAY'S MEALS

Breakfast:	Lunch:	Dinner:
Breakfast Salad (page 130)	*Leftover* Sausage & Spinach "Polenta" Bowl	*Leftover* Super Garlic Meatballs with Fried Rice

Snack(s): Two-Bite Chocolate Cream Pies

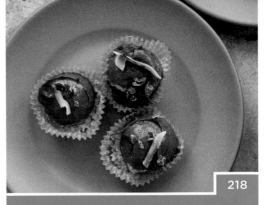

218

TODAY'S RECIPE
Two-Bite Chocolate Cream Pies

TODAY'S CHECKLIST

☐ **Post to social media** using the hashtag #21DSD about your experience. Tell us about your transformation, whether it's emotional, mental, or physical—or all of the above!

☐ **Complete your post-detox assessment on the next 2 pages!** Use the past 21 days of journal responses to remind yourself of your progress (and ups and downs!) along the way.

" *I did it! 21 days no sugar! I'm so glad I did this. I've learned to look at every label. I love vegetables! Before this I would fill up on carbs and throw out the veggies. Now I could eat a meal of all veggies. I'm planning to stay on this road with a keto lifestyle. I could have never done it without this detox!* "

— Christi S. (21DSD Community Member)

SLEEP TIME & QUALITY

to bed last night _____

woke up today_____

☐ excellent   ☐ fair

☐ good   ☐ poor

✎ NOTES ABOUT TODAY

Right now, I'm most proud of myself for... _____

_____

_____

_____

Something I accomplished during the detox that I couldn't before was... _____

_____

_____

_____

EXERCISE

time _____

_____

type _____

_____

I feel... _____

_____

_____

_____

MOOD & ENERGY

☐ excellent   ☐ fair

☐ good   ☐ poor

notes _____

_____

TODAY'S FRUIT

🍎 or 🍌 or 🍊

On these pages, write down your full **21DSD story** by filling in your experience after each of the prompts. Completing these pages is important to rounding out your experience, and it's helpful to have this to refer back to long after you've completed the program. Your own personal lessons are what I most want you to carry forward from your 21DSD experience.

Before the 21DSD, I would describe my eating habits as . . .

_____

_____

_____

_____

_____

_____

Over the course of the last three weeks, I was able to focus on . . .

_____

_____

_____

_____

_____

_____

_____

_____

Three changes I've made to my everyday eating habits regarding food are . . .

_____

_____

_____

_____

_____

_____

_____

Two elements of my overall lifestyle (aside from food choices) that changed while on the 21DSD were . . .

_____

_____

_____

_____

_____

_____

_____

The thing I thought I couldn't do that I did was . . . _____

_____

_____

_____

_____

_____

Positive changes in my life I experienced over the course of the 21DSD were . . . _____

_____

_____

_____

_____

_____

_____

Any other thoughts or feelings you don't want to forget about your 21DSD experience? Write them here.

_____

_____

_____

_____

_____

_____

_____

_____

_____

One person I plan to tell about this program, and who would really do well on it, is . . . ____

_____

_____

_____

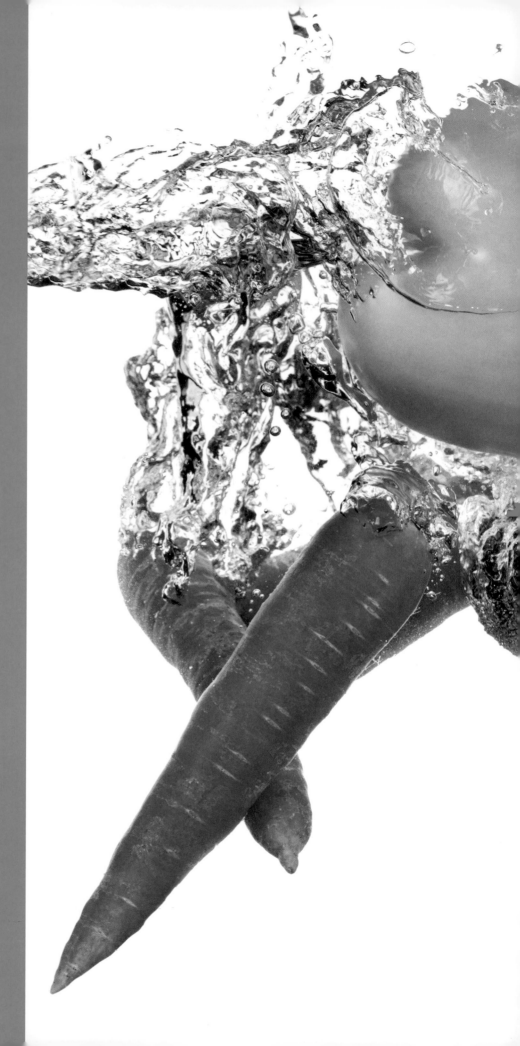

THE
WEEK
AFTER
YOUR
DETOX

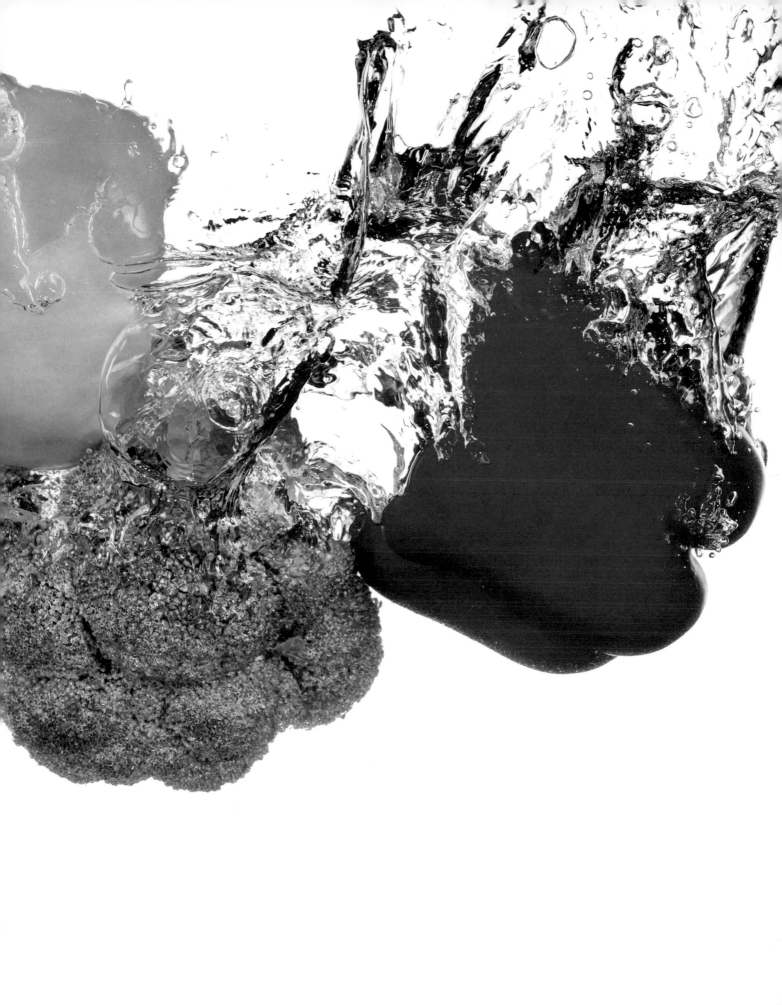

The Dish from Diane

I know how tempting it can be to look at today as a day to reward yourself for completing the 21DSD—likely with food! And, in some ways, that's okay. If you take a moment to reward your hard work and efforts with *healthy* sweet foods, like berries and a bit of some dark chocolate, you're going to feel amazing. Your sense of accomplishment for getting through three weeks will remain, and you'll feel like those naturally sweet berries were special—and that dark chocolate will probably taste sweeter than you remembered! But while an all-out gluten-and-booze bender may *sound* like fun, it isn't the best plan of attack. For your physical and emotional health, it's better to celebrate your 21DSD wrap-up with healthy sweet foods or a non-food reward—a nice manicure, a new kitchen gadget, or even a new healthy-eating cookbook!

TODAY'S CHECKLIST

- [ ] **Reward yourself!** You made it through the 21DSD! Pat yourself on the back and treat yourself to some dark chocolate or a massage or that book you've been wanting to buy.

- [ ] **Reintroduce a food** and track how you respond in the chart on page 91.

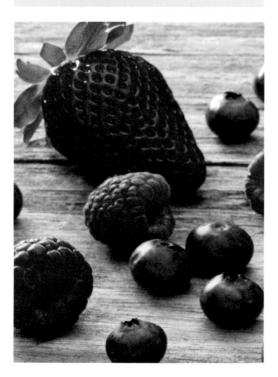

1 DAY Post-Detox

TODAY'S LESSON
Bringing back foods you've missed!

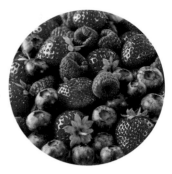

This week is designed to help you transition back to your "normal life" while incorporating what you've learned over the last twenty-one days. The first thing you'll probably want to do is bring back some foods you've been missing. To really get the benefits of the detox, reintroduce foods slowly, over the next seven days. (You are also welcome to continue the reintroduction process *beyond* this post-detox week, as you see fit.)

At right you'll find a list of foods to bring back to your plate, listed in order of when I recommend you reintroduce them (try berries first, for instance). You'll notice that I don't list artificial sweeteners (e.g., aspartame, Splenda, Truvia) or vegetable oils (e.g., canola, soybean, sunflower)—because of their effects on health, I do not recommend consuming those regularly.

So, for example, today you may choose to bring back some berries or sweet fruits like mango or pineapple. In the chart on the facing page, keep notes on how you feel as a result of eating these foods. You may not notice much, or you may notice a lot—it varies a ton from person to person.

Don't reintroduce a new food tomorrow—stick with just what you added today. The reintroduction of a food should be a two-day process, to give you time to respond to each food before adding another. Then, on your "day 24" (three days after your detox), choose the next food you want to reintroduce, like dark chocolate, goat cheese, or white rice, for example. You'll continue this process of adding back a food every other day to allow time for your body to process it and for you to feel the effects of that food.

Depending on the level at which you completed your 21DSD and how you're feeling with the changes you've made, you may decide to slowly reintroduce a lot of different foods, or you may choose to keep most of them off of your plate going forward. Many people opt to follow a gluten-free, grain-free, or more Paleo way of eating following the 21-Day Sugar Detox, though that certainly isn't required. If you'd like some more detailed steps for following a Paleo diet, I highly recommend you grab a copy of my first book, *Practical Paleo*. It includes meal plans if you'd like that guidance.

LEVELS	FOOD
All	**Berries:** strawberries, raspberries, blueberries, etc.
All	**Sweet fruits:** mango, pineapple, peaches, oranges, etc.
All	**Dark chocolate**, 80% cacao and above
Level 3	**Goat or sheep dairy** (try before moving to cow dairy)
Level 3	**Cow dairy:** Start with hard cheeses, then soft cheeses, then cream or milk
Levels 2 & 3	**Gluten-free whole grains** like rice, oats, or quinoa
All	**Gluten-free grain flours** like rice flour, corn flour, or other gluten-free flour blends or foods made with them (gluten-free bread, etc.)
All	**Gluten-containing whole grains or grain flours**, like wheat, barley, or rye (generally not recommended)
All	**Soy-based foods** like tofu, edamame, or soy milk (generally not recommended)

DATE:	Before eating
Food / Food group:	*Describe how you*
ENERGY	*pretty good*
MOOD/EMOTIONS	*even*
SKIN	*clear*
DIGESTION & ELIMINATION	*normal*
SLEEP	*sound*
HORMONES	*seem good*
OTHER	*feeling good*

THE 21-DAY SUGAR DETOX FOOD REINTRODUCTION ASSESSMENT

DATE: Food / Food group:	Before eating	Immediately after eating	1–2 hours after eating	4–8 hours after eating	The day after eating
	Describe how you feel before and after eating this food using general terms like poor, fair, good, great; then add description and detail				
ENERGY					
MOOD/EMOTIONS					
SKIN					
DIGESTION & ELIMINATION					
SLEEP					
HORMONES					
OTHER					

The Dish from Diane

Dying to reintroduce wine? Or maybe some gluten-filled foods? Please be very slow and deliberate about these choices. I don't want you to throw away the hard work you've done in dropping them cold turkey without thinking hard about it and evaluating how they really affect you, physically and emotionally. Wine and gluten-containing foods specifically can be problematic, much more so than sweet fruit, because they can become a crutch—something that we turn to when what we really need is emotional support. Be thoughtful about reintroducing them, and pay close attention to how you feel both physically and emotionally during and after consuming each food you reintroduce. Remember, the long-term goal of the 21DSD is to help you learn how your body feels with and without these foods so that you can make healthy choices for a lifetime—so instead of feeling like you constantly need to come back to the detox as your baseline, you can find your own new "normal." More on this in tomorrow's lesson!

TODAY'S CHECKLIST

☐ **Take notes** on how you're doing with the food you reintroduced yesterday, using the chart on page 91.

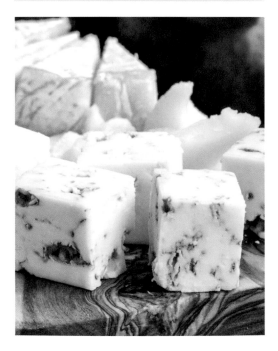

TODAY'S LESSON

Reintroduction reactions

This week is all about assessment! Taking a slow, strategic approach to reintroducing non-21DSD foods will help you make a smooth transition to a sustainable healthy-eating lifestyle instead of feeling like you are always either "on the plan" or "off the plan." It also helps you find out which foods you're better off cutting out completely. We all want to find that balance that works for us in the long term, where we can make healthy choices the vast majority of the time without getting derailed when we occasionally make a choice that isn't as healthy. When you know how your body responds to certain foods, it's easier to navigate which choices are worth it and which aren't.

For example, I don't experience any digestive or skin-related issues as a result of eating goat and sheep dairy, but I do when I eat cow dairy. So while I avoid cow dairy, I actually enjoy my meals more when I add small amounts of goat and sheep dairy to my plate—it feels less restrictive, so I don't feel like I want to rebel by eating unhealthy foods.

Possible reactions to newly reintroduced foods can include low energy, fatigue, brain fog, feeling low or unhappy, skin reactions (acne or a rash), digestive upset (gas, bloating, diarrhea, or constipation), trouble sleeping, increased menstrual symptoms, or a sense that something is "off," that you're not quite yourself.

The self-awareness that comes from testing how you feel when you eat certain foods will fuel a sense of peace and calm around eating off-plan foods—you won't be worried about possible effects or feel guilty, because you already know what works for you.

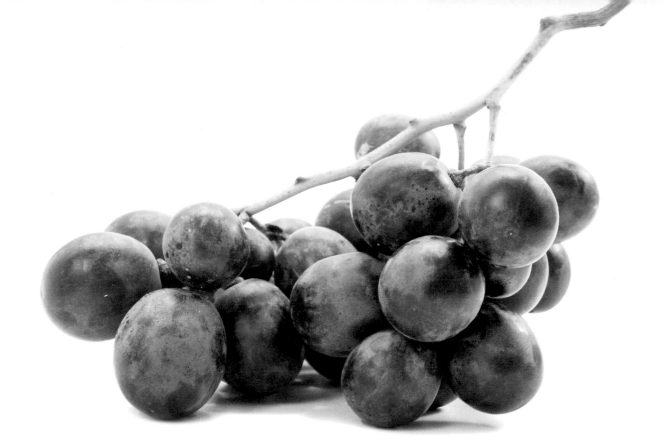

✎ NOTES ABOUT TODAY

A success I had today was... _____

_____

_____

_____

A challenging moment today was... _____

_____

_____

_____

Something that surprised me today was... _____

_____

_____

_____

notes _____

_____

_____

SLEEP TIME & QUALITY

to bed last night _____

woke up today _____

☐ excellent   ☐ fair

☐ good   ☐ poor

EXERCISE

time _____

_____

type _____

_____

MOOD & ENERGY

☐ excellent   ☐ fair

☐ good   ☐ poor

The Dish from Diane

Just because a friend, spouse, or loved one does well with moderation doesn't mean that it's the "right" way to operate. Allow me to give you the space to recognize if you simply do better abstaining from certain foods or activities. For some reason, people don't question it if you don't want to smoke a cigarette just because they're smoking one, but when it comes to a cookie, they can't seem to help trying to persuade you that "just one cookie isn't a big deal." You're allowed to decide what feels best for you—whether that means enjoying something in moderation or not!

TODAY'S CHECKLIST

☐ **Reintroduce a food** and track how you respond in the chart on page 95.

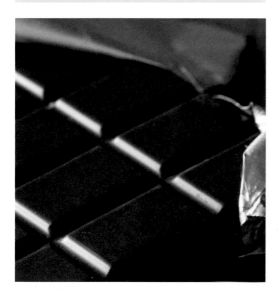

TODAY'S LESSON
Everything in moderation?

We've all heard that the best diet advice is "everything in moderation." (You may have heard it from friends and family during your detox—it's a common criticism.) But this isn't always true, not for everyone and not for every food. Some people do well with the concept of "everything in moderation," but others truly do not.

For many people, one serving (or even one bite) of a tempting but unhealthy food will send them into an all-day—or even all-week or longer—tailspin. Some people do just fine having a small bite or two of something sweet, but others feel like it's all or nothing and do better without a bite at all. Neither approach is wrong, they're simply different. We all need to figure out what works for us, then proceed accordingly.

I'll also note that the idea of having some foods in moderation while avoiding others entirely is completely valid. You may find that you don't have an issue eating a couple of squares of dark chocolate (a lovely post-detox food and a nice occasional treat), while someone else might feel compelled to eat the whole bar. At the same time, you may find that dried mango (another great post-detox food choice) goes down far too easily for you and you can't seem to stop eating it once you start.

So, for each of us, it's important to find out whether we tend to do better with moderation or not and if there are certain foods that we just can't eat in moderation. Then proceed accordingly.

> "Life isn't about finding yourself. Life is about creating yourself."
>
> — George Bernard Shaw

THE 21-DAY SUGAR DETOX FOOD REINTRODUCTION ASSESSMENT

DATE:	Before eating	Immediately after eating	1–2 hours after eating	4–8 hours after eating	The day after eating
Food / Food group:	*Describe how you feel before and after eating this food using general terms like poor, fair, good, great; then add description and detail*				
ENERGY					
MOOD/EMOTIONS					
SKIN					
DIGESTION & ELIMINATION					
SLEEP					
HORMONES					
OTHER					

✎ NOTES ABOUT TODAY

A success I had today was... _____

_____

_____

A challenging moment today was... _____

_____

_____

_____

Something that surprised me today was... _____

_____

_____

_____

notes _____

_____

SLEEP TIME & QUALITY
to bed last night _____
woke up today _____

☐ excellent   ☐ fair
☐ good   ☐ poor

EXERCISE
time _____
_____
type _____
_____

MOOD & ENERGY
☐ excellent   ☐ fair
☐ good   ☐ poor

TODAY'S CHECKLIST

- [ ] **Take notes** on how you're doing with the food you reintroduced yesterday, using the chart on page 95.

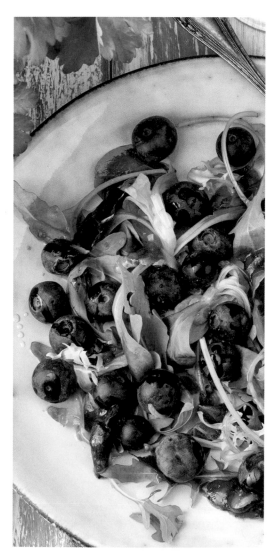

TODAY'S LESSON
Finding *your* new normal, part 1

For the last three weeks, you've had strict rules around what not to eat. For many of you, the idea that there are no longer rules hanging over your head may leave you wondering, "Now what? How do I move forward to create a new normal?" Or maybe you're feeling relieved—you've learned something and you have an idea of how to build your post-detox plate to include some non-21DSD foods while incorporating what you now know about yourself.

Since we all have different personalities and handle rules and expectations differently, we actually can't all move forward from the 21DSD in the same way! I know this seems tricky, but I'll give you some practical ways to figure out what feels best for you.

Scenario 1: "My rules, your rules, either works for me!"
Post-21DSD, you feel like you've learned how you want to move ahead by incorporating some of the rules that work for you, and it feels like it'll be hard to maintain the lifestyle you want to without the rules of the program to hold you accountable. You may not struggle to maintain healthy habits when you're not "on a plan" anymore.

> **Your best bet:** Decide which elements of the program you'll abide by and which you feel you can happily bend. For example, perhaps you'll continue to avoid soy and gluten, but you'll add back in a daily serving or two of berries or other sweet fruits. This way, you can stick to what you've found works for you while you take what you learned on the program into your everyday life.

Scenario 2: "I do better with someone else's rules."
Post-21DSD, you feel free, which is sort of nice, but you're almost *too* free! Without the structure of the rules of the program, you feel like you don't quite know how to achieve the balance you can and want to achieve. You may feel like not being on a plan is truly causing a lot of stress for you.

> **Your best bet:** Collaborate with some friends or accountability partners to help maintain your healthy habits. It can certainly be your spouse, roommate, or other friend or loved one, but it could also be a buddy you've made online or someone you keep in touch with via text. Plan to check in when you aren't sure if you're making the healthiest decision. If you set up this accountability, it'll be a lot easier to maintain your healthy habits.

Don't recognize yourself in either of these descriptions? I'll look at two more common scenarios in tomorrow's lesson.

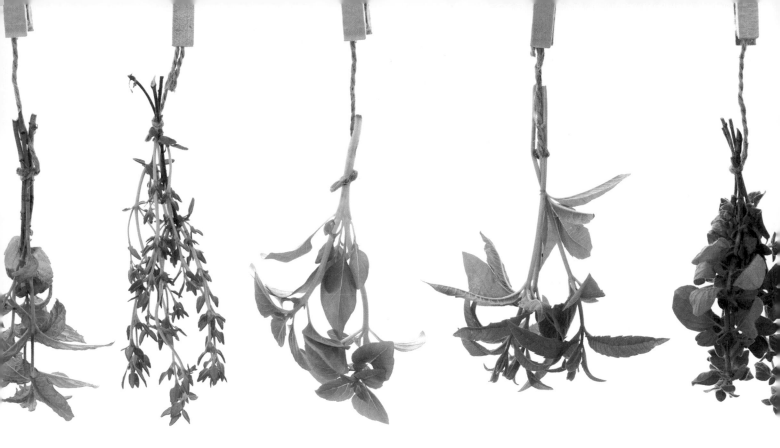

✎ NOTES ABOUT TODAY

A success I had today was... _____

_____

_____

_____

_____

A challenging moment today was... _____

_____

_____

_____

Something that surprised me today was... _____

_____

_____

_____

notes _____

_____

_____

SLEEP TIME & QUALITY

to bed last night _____

woke up today _____

☐ excellent   ☐ fair

☐ good   ☐ poor

EXERCISE

time _____

_____

type _____

_____

MOOD & ENERGY

☐ excellent   ☐ fair

☐ good   ☐ poor

TODAY'S CHECKLIST

- [ ] **Reintroduce a food** and track how you respond in the chart on page 99.

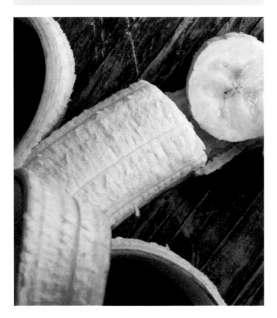

> "You become what you think about most of the time."
>
> — Brian Tracy

TODAY'S LESSON
Finding *your* new normal, part 2

Yesterday we looked at two common approaches to life post-detox. Today we'll look at two more.

Scenario 3: "Why would I keep following your rules when I can make my own rules now?"

Post-21DSD, you feel glad that you did it—it was worth it and based on sound reasoning—but now you're unsure *why* you'd continue many of the habits you changed while on the program. Yes, they made sense for the purposes of the 21DSD, but you wonder if all of those rules and restrictions really make sense for you in the long term.

> **Your best bet:** Decide which healthy habits you want to stick to and continue to read up on why avoiding sugar and foods like wheat and soy, for example, is something worth perpetuating. I highly recommend grabbing a copy of *Practical Paleo,* second edition, and reading the first part of the book; it'll answer all of your questions about why you'd eat primarily real, whole foods for a lifetime.

Scenario 4: "I go by how I feel. I don't do things because of rules, whether my own or yours."

Post-21DSD, you feel proud that you stuck with the program as you said you would, and it wasn't because anyone else wanted you to. The rules of the program felt neither overly strict nor overly easy, because you really chose to be "in it" for the three weeks. Now you're wondering what you really want to do moving forward. *Do I want to eat this way? Do I want to use some of these tools and not others? Which parts of this program feel right for me long-term and which don't?*

> **Your best bet:** Identify what it is about completing this program and eating healthfully in general makes you feel like *you.* Is it that your energy is higher, and a high-energy person is who you are (and want to be)? Does making healthy choices make you feel like you're putting your best foot forward in the world? For me, knowing that I'm a healthy person who eats mostly real, whole foods keeps me grounded in a lifestyle that's largely sugar-free, while I am able to sometimes enjoy a treat without going out of control.

THE 21-DAY SUGAR DETOX FOOD REINTRODUCTION ASSESSMENT

DATE: Food / Food group:	Before eating	Immediately after eating	1–2 hours after eating	4–8 hours after eating	The day after eating
	Describe how you feel before and after eating this food using general terms like poor, fair, good, great; then add description and detail				
ENERGY					
MOOD/EMOTIONS					
SKIN					
DIGESTION & ELIMINATION					
SLEEP					
HORMONES					
OTHER					

✎ NOTES ABOUT TODAY

A success I had today was... _____

_____

_____

_____

A challenging moment today was... _____

_____

_____

_____

Something that surprised me today was... _____

_____

_____

_____

notes _____

_____

SLEEP TIME & QUALITY

to bed last night _____

woke up today _____

- [ ] excellent
- [ ] good
- [ ] fair
- [ ] poor

EXERCISE

time _____

_____

type _____

_____

MOOD & ENERGY

- [ ] excellent
- [ ] good
- [ ] fair
- [ ] poor

TODAY'S CHECKLIST

- [ ] **Take notes** on how you're doing with the food you reintroduced yesterday, using the chart on page 99.

> **"What you do every day matters more than what you do once in a while."**
>
> — Gretchen Rubin

TODAY'S LESSON

Short-term strategies for balancing healthy eating and now-and-then indulgences

Integrating healthy choices into daily life can look different for everyone, so here are a few ways to move through an indulgent moment, a meal, or a day or two of indulgence without guilt, shame, or spiraling out of control. There's no need to give a treat power over you, especially after twenty-one days of not eating it! *You* have the power to make the choice.

In a moment

In this case, a moment can be considered one treat or time when you're offered one. There are a couple of ways to approach these moments. For one, you could simply say, "No, thank you," and pass on the treat. Or take a few bites, and if it isn't delicious, then put it down. There's no need to feel FOMO (fear of missing out) over a cupcake now and then. You can literally have a cupcake *anytime* you want.

Now, on the flip side, if you truly want the cupcake, then just eat it, enjoy the moment, and move on with your life. The next choice you make can easily be a healthy one. There's no reason for enjoying a cupcake to spiral into a train of guilt and shame about the choice to eat it.

I'm giving you permission right now: eat the cupcake, then move on with healthy choices. End of story.

For a meal

Maybe it's your birthday, or maybe you're eating at a really great restaurant, and what you want to enjoy isn't as healthy as it could be. Again, you have a choice to make. Decide that your meals before and after will be healthy ones, go enjoy your meal, then return to your healthy choices after—no guilt or shame. Make the choice to enjoy it and move on.

For a day or two

Maybe you've got some work travel coming up, or maybe you have visitors in town and you're dining out more often than usual. Have groceries ready for when the time frame ends—at least one or two sources of protein, some salad greens, or maybe some frozen cauliflower rice and some eggs. When you're ready to return to your usual routine, your house will be already stocked with healthy food, so you can bounce right back into the swing of things.

On a vacation

While it's not a good idea to be on the 21DSD while you're on vacation, after your detox, you can still enjoy a vacation in a healthy way.

Start your mornings off right. Eat a breakfast with quality protein and healthy fats—eggs, meat, avocado—and some vegetables. Try to avoid a sugary breakfast, aside from perhaps some fresh fruit. Then, as your day unfolds, make choices that feel special and worth it for your vacation. If you come across a local delicacy, enjoy it. There's no way I'd encourage you to travel to Italy and *not* try some handmade pasta with fresh Parmigiano-Reggiano, unless you already know that you don't feel well when you eat gluten and dairy.

There's no need to feel bad about these choices. Simply make them, enjoy the food, enjoy your new experiences, and—you guessed it! — bounce back to healthy eating when you get home.

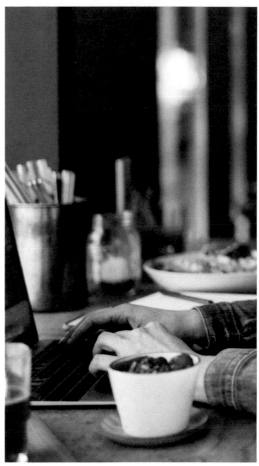

✎ NOTES ABOUT TODAY

A success I had today was... _____

_____

_____

_____

A challenging moment today was... _____

_____

_____

_____

Something that surprised me today was... _____

_____

_____

_____

notes _____

_____

SLEEP TIME & QUALITY

to bed last night _____

woke up today_____

☐ excellent   ☐ fair

☐ good   ☐ poor

EXERCISE

time _____

type _____

MOOD & ENERGY

☐ excellent   ☐ fair

☐ good   ☐ poor

TODAY'S CHECKLIST

- [ ] **Reintroduce a food** and track how you respond in the chart on page 103.

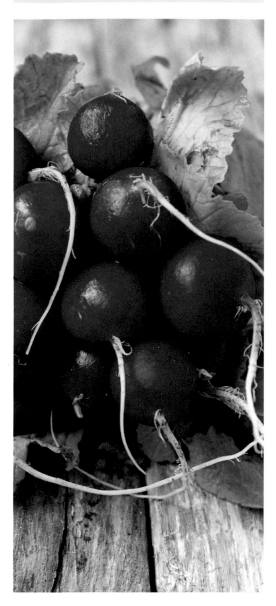

> **"The beautiful thing about learning is that no one can take it away from you."**
>
> — B.B. King

TODAY'S LESSON

The long game: Finding what works for you in the long term

In this case, "long term" means beyond this post-detox week, and beyond the next month. I don't expect you to jump on and off the 21DSD for years and years. I want you to find what works for you for the next year and the years that follow—a sustainable long-term diet and lifestyle that work *specifically for you.*

This can seem daunting, but the answer truly lies in living out the coming weeks, months, and even years. Most who have come to a real-food way of eating—eschewing refined grains, sugars, and seed oils in favor of more colorful, fresher, and more vibrant and nutritious foods—didn't land on their perfect diet in three weeks or even three months. The 21DSD can help kick-start this process and make it easier to get to a place where sugar doesn't run your life, but you need to live through more time after this program to see how it will all play out for you. You need to experience the ups and downs of eating foods that work well for you, physically and emotionally, and some that don't, in order to make informed decisions on how you want to eat as your life goes on. By being mindful of how your choices feel for your body and for your mindset, you will figure out which foods are worth it for you to indulge in and which aren't.

Here's an example: my husband loves craft beer. The problem: craft beer doesn't love him back. He's gluten intolerant, and gluten is in all beer (unless it is specifically made to be gluten-free). If he drinks beer (or eats any gluten), he gets an itchy rash on his elbows. He instantly knows when he's eaten something with gluten, and it causes enough discomfort for him that it's not worth it. But he doesn't want to live a life without the pleasure he derives from a fermented, alcoholic, beer-type beverage on occasion. So, how does he enjoy a drink now and then? He's found something that works better for him than beer: hard cider. Finding new craft ciders to try has even become a bit of a hobby for him. This is how he's translated a dietary lesson into a lifestyle choice that works for him for the long term.

Another example: I love sweets. The problem: well, you know by now that sweets don't truly love *anyone* back. At least, not the kind I used to eat. And in the amounts I used to eat. And with the frequency with which I used to eat them. Once upon a time I frequently indulged in extremely sweet candy. I'm talking the *really* sugary kind. If it was gummy and sour, I was in! But over time, by cutting sugar out, then reintroducing it, then cutting it out again, I was able to both know and *feel* the impact that those junky sugars have on my body.

So, how do I live my life day to day, knowing that I love those candies but also knowing that they aren't welcome in my diet? I replace them with their natural counterparts: fresh berries, dried mango (an excellent gummy-candy replacement—sweet and sour and chewy all at once!), and even, maybe once a year, a very small portion of organic sour candy. I enjoy dark chocolate several times a week, and maybe once a month I bake a gluten-free treat.

These are just a couple of examples, and you can read lots more at 21DSD.com/stories.

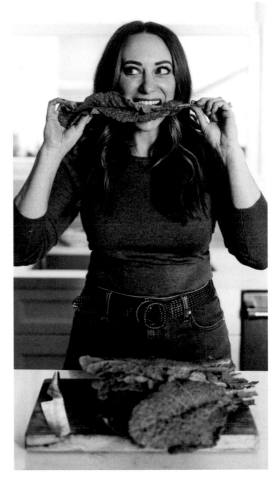

Personal experience is key. A book can tell you why sugar, refined foods, and gluten aren't going to work well for you. A friend can tell you that eating this way or that way worked wonders for them. Your doctor can tell you that you need to stop eating sugar or drinking alcohol. But to build a lifestyle that works for you, you must experience how you feel without certain foods in your diet, then bring them back and pay close attention to how you feel (as you've started doing in this post-detox week), then remove them again.

I want you to be able to enjoy less-than-healthy foods you love now and then, without shame or guilt. And if you're not there yet—if indulging once a week or once a month makes you feel out of control—that's okay. Wait until you feel that you can eat those foods, go right back to your healthy habits afterward, and don't feel shame about the decision you made to have a treat and get on with your life.

THE 21-DAY SUGAR DETOX FOOD REINTRODUCTION ASSESSMENT

DATE:	Before eating	Immediately after eating	1-2 hours after eating	4-8 hours after eating	The day after eating
Food / Food group:	*Describe how you feel before and after eating this food using general terms like poor, fair, good, great; then add description and detail*				
ENERGY					
MOOD/EMOTIONS					
SKIN					
DIGESTION & ELIMINATION					
SLEEP					
HORMONES					
OTHER					

USEFUL GUIDES

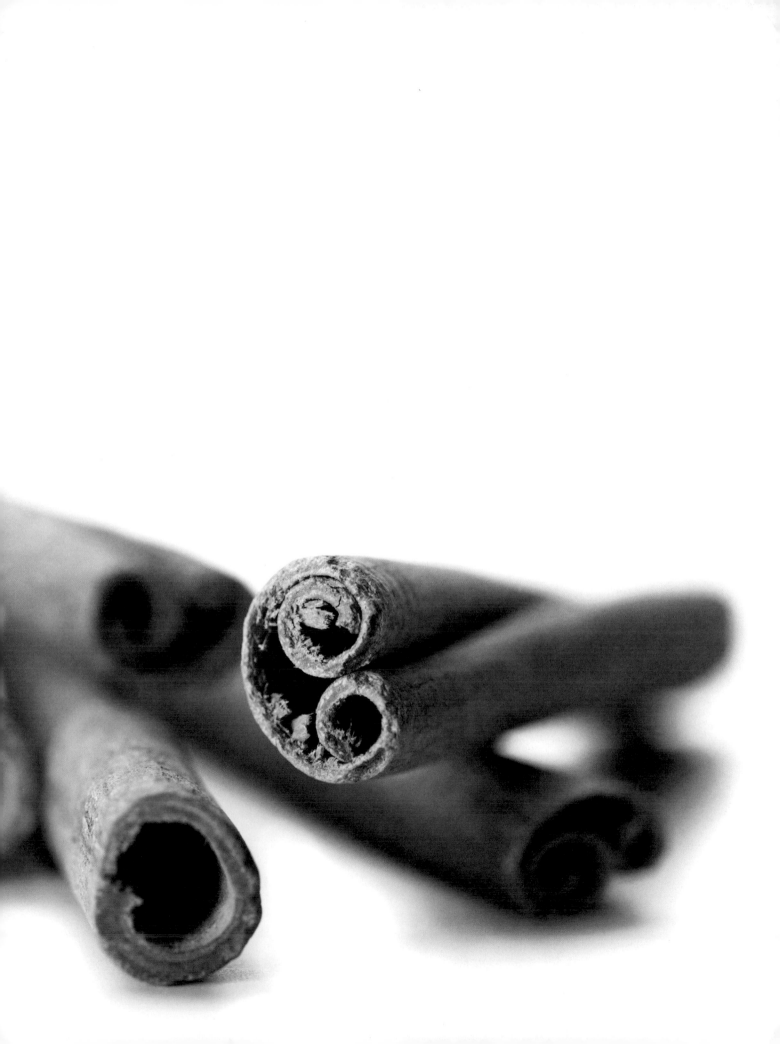

GUIDE TO
HELPFUL SUPPLEMENTS

You are absolutely not required to take any supplements while on the 21-Day Sugar Detox. However, many participants do find them extremely helpful. This guide will help you decide if any of these may be helpful for you.

I always recommend that you try natural, food-based approaches to curbing cravings before you look to herbal or vitamin and mineral supplements for support. Two great solutions are:

- **Lemon water** (sometimes with L-glutamine added; see below). Hydrating with a hint of flavor from lemon or other citrus can help with that urge to grab something sweet.

- **Herbal teas** (sometimes with a touch of full-fat coconut milk added)—more details below

I've listed the supplements here in the order that I suggest trying them. Cinnamon is the #1 supplemental super-spice I recommend adding to your food while on the 21DSD.

If water and tea don't lessen your cravings, you can try a few different herbs and supplements. Everybody is unique and will respond differently to them, but they're all pretty mild and should have only beneficial effects in the moderate dosages recommended here.

With all of the supplements, more does not necessarily mean better. It is always best to start out at a low dose for a few days so that you can see how your system responds.

Helpful Supplements for the 21-Day Sugar Detox

HERBAL TEA

What is it? Blends of caffeine-free herbs that can be steeped to create a hot or cold beverage. Herbal teas support different body systems, so read the descriptions to find out more. That said, tea's "medicinal" properties are typically pretty mild, so you needn't be concerned that a tea has specific properties if you love to drink it simply for its flavor. I love the Traditional Medicinals brand of organic teas. Here are some varieties that you may want to try: ginger, peppermint, licorice root.

What does it do? Herbal teas provide a healthy replacement for the habit of having something sweet after a meal, or for an afternoon or evening snack you may reach for out of boredom, or simply for a craving.

When should I take it? Herbal teas are caffeine-free, so you can enjoy them any time of the day. If you are enjoying licorice root tea or if it is an ingredient in your tea blend, drink it only before 3 p.m., as it can have a stimulating effect.

How much should I take? You can drink as many cups of herbal tea as you like! Keep in mind that it is often better to use one tea bag for multiple cups of tea so that the strength is diluted over time, instead of drinking very potent tea all day.

CINNAMON

What is it? An aromatic spice.

What does it do? Cinnamon helps regulate blood sugar while creating a taste effect that you're eating something sweet, giving the satisfaction of a treat without triggering your body's sweet-taste response. Cinnamon slows the rate at which the stomach empties, which helps keep blood sugar from spiking after meals.

When should I take it? Feel free to enjoy cinnamon on foods at any time of day. Many of the treat recipes in this book include cinnamon.

How much should I take? You can add as much cinnamon as you like to the foods you eat, or sprinkle it in tea or coffee. Add up to 1 1/2 teaspoons to full-fat coconut milk- or almond milk–based smoothies following the recipes in this book. You may also decide to make one of the sweetener-free treat recipes and add cinnamon according to your taste preferences. Cinnamon can also be paired with other flavorings, like curry or chili powder, to season meats—especially pork chops, ground beef, or lamb—and create a sweet-and-savory dish.

L-GLUTAMINE

What is it? An amino acid. Dietary sources of L-glutamine include high-protein foods like beef, chicken, fish, and eggs. This supplement tends to be far more effective at battling cravings when taken in conjunction with a diet rich in these foods.

What does it do? L-glutamine supports the repair of the gut lining (small intestine) and improves gut function, which will always help regulate your body's systems, including metabolism and cravings. It also helps reduce sugar cravings by providing energy to cells.

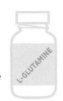

When should I take it? Between meals, beginning as early and ending as late in the day as you like.

How much should I take? In powder form, 2 to 4 grams in water up to twice a day. If you experience any constipation after adding L-glutamine to your daily routine, stop taking it until your eliminations become regular again, then resume it at half the dose.

MAGNESIUM

What is it? A mineral. Dietary sources include kelp, pumpkin seeds, sunflower seeds, spinach, broccoli, Swiss chard, salmon, oysters, halibut, scallops, dried herbs, and bone broth.

What does it do? Magnesium plays a role in more than 300 enzymatic processes in the body, and it has a particularly important role in powering cellular energy production. It also helps insulin take action appropriately; blood sugar management is much easier when you get enough magnesium.

When should I take it? Magnesium can be taken at any time of day, but it can have a relaxing effect, so you may find that taking it in the evening after dinner is ideal.

How much should I take? *Option 1:* 300 to 600 milligrams a day of Natural Calm unflavored powdered drink mix (magnesium citrate). You can use 1/2 teaspoon to begin and go up from there if needed. People who weigh less than 130 pounds should take the lower end of the range. If you experience loose stools after taking a dose, take less the next time. Take this supplement no more than once per day. I recommend mixing it with lemon water.

Option 2: 300 to 600 milligrams a day of magnesium glycinate or magnesium malate in capsule form.

CHROMIUM

What is it? A mineral that can be found on shelves as chromium picolinate, chromium polynicotinate, and chromium chelavite. Dietary sources include eggs, onions, romaine lettuce, ripe tomatoes, liver, peppers, green apples with peel, and sea vegetables like nori (dried seaweed paper), kelp, and dulse.

What does it do? Chromium helps increase insulin sensitivity, which affects how well your body regulates its blood sugar levels. According to naturopath Michael Murray, "Chromium supplementation is indicated in both diabetes and hypoglycemia because of its ability to improve blood sugar control."

When should I take it? With meals; if you are taking one or two doses a day, take them with breakfast and lunch and not with dinner.

How much should I take? 200 micrograms one to three times a day (a total of 200 to 600 micrograms).

B VITAMINS

What is it? Water-soluble vitamins. Dietary sources of B vitamins include liver, dairy (if you are eating raw/unpasteurized or organic full-fat dairy), leafy greens, eggs, and meats (which mainly provide B12).

What does it do? B vitamins play an important role in the complex process of cell metabolism. They help combat fatigue and are often lacking in the diet.

When should I take it? Take vitamin B complex with breakfast and lunch. B vitamins often give the sensation of an energy boost, so it's best to avoid them in the evening.

How much should I take? 100 milligrams twice a day of vitamin B complex.

GYMNEMA

What is it? An herb also known as gymnema sylvestre. You may find it in capsule, tablet, powder, or liquid form. If you can find the leaves, you may chew on them or steep them with your herbal tea.

What does it do? Gymnema can reduce the taste of sugar when it's placed in the mouth, thereby assisting in limiting your sugar cravings.

When should I take it? Anytime you anticipate a craving, or whenever you drink an herbal tea from which you don't want to experience sweetness.

How much should I take? Follow the dosage instructions on the package you buy and start out slowly. Try one dose and go from there based on how you feel.

MORE TIPS & TRICKS
Smart Dining on the 21DSD

1. Think ahead and don't arrive starving. Eat a small snack of some nuts or nut butter, or even a few bites of avocado or leftover meat, before you head out the door.

2. Preview the restaurant's menu online before you go.

3. Check out reviews from other diners on a site like Yelp or TripAdvisor (especially when traveling).

4. Pass on the bread basket—it'll keep temptation away! Ask for sliced veggies or olives instead.

5. Either skip the appetizers or opt for a salad starter.

6. Entrées are easy. While finger food is often breaded, fried, or otherwise carb-loaded, entrées that are made of simpler ingredients can be easy to find.

7. Look for grilled, broiled, or baked options. These typically aren't breaded, so they'll be safer bets for your detox. But ask the server for details on how things are prepared; they're used to questions! Be polite, but get the answers you need.

8. Make substitutions. If a meal comes with french fries, bread, or pasta, simply ask that the kitchen either leave it off of the plate or substitute some vegetables instead.

9. (AT PARTIES) Before you go, ask the host what they plan on serving, so you know what to expect.

10. (AT PARTIES) Bring a dish or two that you know you can enjoy and that will satisfy your hunger. The host will be happy to have the contribution, and you'll be glad to know that you won't be hungry all night if they're serving only foods that you aren't currently eating.

For a guide to what to eat at specific restaurant chains on the 21DSD, visit 21DSD.com/guides

AMERICAN FOOD

AVOID: Fried foods, anything breaded, sandwiches, wraps, and premade dressings.

ENJOY: Bunless or lettuce-wrapped burgers and salads with lemon or vinegar and olive oil. Entrées with grilled, steamed, or baked proteins and vegetables without sauces. Add olive oil, butter, vinegar, and lemon to season.

CHINESE FOOD

AVOID: Unless you know the restaurant well enough to make special requests for no MSG and only sauces without sugar, it's best to avoid Chinese food. Many of the sauces contain hidden sweeteners and soy.

INDIAN FOOD

AVOID: Skip the naan and rice. Ask about flour/gluten in sauces and spice rubs.

ENJOY: Meats and veggies that are grilled or roasted and not drowning in sauces. Tandoori meats are often marinated in yogurt, so they're okay on Levels 1 and 2, but not on Level 3.

ITALIAN FOOD & PIZZA

AVOID: Bread, pasta, and breaded meats. Ask about sauces and preparation of items (meatballs often contain breadcrumbs). There is simply no great way to enjoy a 21DSD version of pizza while dining out.

ENJOY: Broiled chicken, fish, shrimp, or other protein with red sauce and veggies or salad on the side. If you're craving pizza, make pizza with a cauliflower or almond meal crust. (Omit the cheese if you are on Level 3.)

JAPANESE FOOD

AVOID: Rice (white and brown) is typically flavored with vinegar, which is okay, and sugar, which is not. Also avoid anything fried or tempura-battered, imitation crab, and most sauces. For Level 1, you can technically have some rice, but I would still avoid it.

ENJOY: Sashimi or broiled fish; just be sure to ask about sauces used and avoid soy sauce. Ask for a side of daikon radish to eat with your fish; most restaurants have it.

MEXICAN FOOD

AVOID: Tortilla shells and chips (both corn and flour), beans, and rice (or eat limited portions per Level 1 & 2 guidelines). Vegetarians: Have some beans but go lightly on the rice per your daily portions.

ENJOY: Meat, salsa, and guacamole—often you can ask for these ingredients to be placed over a salad or with vegetables. Ask for raw celery or carrots to dip into guacamole. Ask for a side of vegetables to add to your entrée.

THAI FOOD

AVOID: Sauces that contain sugar (ask about ingredients). Also avoid noodles, Thai iced tea (typically presweetened), and desserts. For Level 1, you can have your included portion of daily rice.

ENJOY: Chicken satay (typically okay) or a curry dish or other coconut milk–based dish without rice. Order extra steamed vegetables.

GUIDE TO HIDDEN SUGARS

While on the 21DSD, all the forms of sugar and sweeteners listed here are out! Always turn packages around to read ingredients. If any of the sweeteners listed below are in the ingredients, that food is out for your detox.^

Note that we are not talking about naturally occurring sugars in foods like yogurt (from natural lactose) or 21DSD-friendly fruits—we're talking about added sweeteners. Also note that seeing grams of sugar in the Nutrition Facts is not the same as finding hidden or added sugar in a product.

^ The two exceptions to the rule to avoid foods with these sweeteners are bacon/cured meats and kombucha. See page 126 for more details on bacon and cured meats.

NATURAL SWEETENERS*

Brown sugar	Date sugar	Maple syrup
Cane juice	Date syrup	Molasses
Cane juice crystals	Dates	Monk fruit
	Fruit juice	Palm sugar
Cane sugar	Fruit juice concentrate	Raw sugar
Coconut nectar		Stevia (green leaf or extract)
Coconut sugar/ crystals	Honey	
	Luo han guo	Turbinado sugar

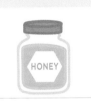

Recommended for using in very limited quantities after your 21DSD.

NATURALLY DERIVED SWEETENERS

Agave	Demerara sugar	Lactose	Sugar alcohols (for example, erythritol, maltitol, mannitol, xylitol; words ending in -ol)
Agave nectar	Dextran	Levulose	
Barley malt	Dextrose	Light brown sugar	
Beet sugar	Diastase		
Brown rice syrup	Diastatic malt	Malt syrup	
Buttered syrup	Ethyl maltol	Maltitol	Swerve (brand name for a sugar alcohol blend)
Carob syrup	Fructose	Maltodextrin	
Corn syrup	Glucose / glucose solids	Maltose	
Corn syrup solids		Mannitol	
	Golden sugar	Muscovado	Tagatose (Tagatesse, Nutrilatose)
	Golden syrup	Refiner's syrup	
	Grape sugar	Sorbitol	Treacle
	High-fructose corn syrup	Sorghum syrup	Yellow sugar
	Invert sugar	Sucrose	Xylitol

ARTIFICIAL SWEETENERS

Acesulfame K / acesulfame potassium (Sweet One, Sunett)

Aspartame (Equal, NutraSweet)

Saccharine (Sweet'N Low)

Stevia, white/bleached (Truvia, Sun Crystals)

Sucralose (Splenda)

AFTER THE DETOX

How It's Made
The more highly refined a sweetener is, the worse it is for your body. For example, high-fructose corn syrup (HFCS) and artificial sweeteners are modern, factory-made products. Honey, maple syrup, green leaf stevia (dried leaves made into powder), and molasses are all much less processed and have been made for hundreds of years. In the case of honey, almost no processing is necessary. As a result, I vote for raw, organic, local honey as the ideal natural sweetener after your 21DSD.

Where It's Used
This is a reality check. When you read the ingredients in packaged, processed foods, it becomes obvious that most of them use highly refined, low-quality sweeteners. Food manufacturers even hide sugar in foods that you didn't think were sweet! Many foods that have been made low-fat or non-fat have added sweeteners or artificial sweeteners—avoid these products!

How Your Body Processes It
Your body does not metabolize all sugar the same way. Interestingly enough, sweeteners like HFCS and agave nectar were viewed as better options for diabetics for quite some time because both are high in fructose, which is processed by the liver before the sugar hits your bloodstream. This yields a seemingly favorable result on blood sugar levels. However, it's now understood that isolated fructose metabolism is a complicated issue and that taxing the liver excessively with such sweeteners can be quite harmful to your health. Fructose is the primary sugar in all fruit. When eating whole fruit, the micronutrients and fiber content of the fruit actually support proper metabolism and assimilation of the fruit sugar. Whole foods for the win!

GUIDE TO
SIMPLE SWAPS

Replace...	With this...
Bread	→ Lettuce or collard wraps for burgers and deli meats, portobello mushroom slices as buns
Crackers (made from grains)	→ Nut- or seed-based crackers, such as Jilz or GoRaw brands; or use thinly sliced fresh vegetables with dips, etc.
Cereal (made from grains)	→ Banana Vanilla Bean N'Oatmeal (page 146) or Grain-Free Banola (page 147)
Cookies or donuts (made from grains)	→ Not-sweet treats found in this book (pages 216 to 227) or anywhere in the 21DSD family of recipes!
Granola bars (made from grains)	→ Bars made from meats and/or nuts and seeds, such as EPIC brand, or jerky and nuts
Nondairy milks (soy, oat, etc.)	→ Unsweetened nut milks, unsweetened coconut milk yogurts, unsweetened hemp milk. (There are many recipes available online; most store-bought brands have too many additives.) Nut, coconut, and hemp milk–based products are okay if unsweetened.
Pancakes (made from grains)	→ Pumpkin Pancakes (page 149) or almond/coconut flour pancakes
Pasta and noodles (made from grains)	→ Spaghetti squash noodles or zucchini cut with a spiral slicer. Or put sauce and meat over roasted vegetables, like the B3 Bowl (page 152).
Protein powders / **shake mixes with multiple ingredients**	→ Single-ingredient protein powders: collagen peptides, pure grass-fed whey protein, pure egg white protein, or pure hemp protein powder, for example
Soy sauce or tamari	→ Coconut aminos (liquid aminos, a soy-based product, is not the same as coconut aminos)
Sweeteners	→ 21DSD-friendly fruits (see page 20)—they may be cooked or raw

FOR LEVELS 1 & 2

Low-fat & nonfat dairy (milk, cheese, yogurt, etc.)	→ Full-fat dairy (sometimes labeled as 4%): milk, cream, and all cheeses from any animal

FOR LEVELS 2 & 3

Rice	→ Riced cauliflower or shredded potatoes

FOR LEVEL 3

Milk (cow, sheep, goat, soy)	→ Coconut milk (page 243) or almond milk (page 242)
Cheese (cow, sheep, goat, soy)	→ For cooking, depending on the recipe: nutritional yeast (see page 127), roasted garlic, or Cashew "Cheese" Sauce (page 235)
Yogurt (cow, sheep, goat, soy)	→ Homemade coconut milk yogurt (there are many recipes available online; most store-bought brands have too many additives). You can also try getting probiotics in other forms, such as sauerkraut.
Whey protein	→ Egg white protein powder, beef-based protein powder, or collagen peptides

GUIDE TO HEALTHY FATS & OILS

cleaning up your diet by using the right fats & oils is essential to improving your health

which to eat

SATURATED
IDEAL FOR HOT USES

PLANT SOURCES
organic, unrefined forms are ideal

Coconut oil

Palm oil from sustainable sources

ANIMAL SOURCES
pasture-raised/grass-fed & organic sources are ideal

Butter, ghee/clarified butter

Duck fat

Lamb fat

Lard

Schmaltz (chicken fat)

Tallow

UNSATURATED
IDEAL FOR COLD USES

Organic, extra-virgin & cold-pressed forms are ideal

Avocado oil

Nut oils
(walnut, pecan, macadamia)

Olive oil

Sesame oil

Nuts & seeds
(including nut & seed butters)

Flaxseed oil
(higher in polyunsaturated fatty acids, so consume in extremely limited amounts)

NOTE: *Unsaturated fats—often called oils, as listed above—are typically liquid at room temperature and are easily damaged (oxidized) when heat is applied to them. You do not want to consume damaged fats; therefore, cooking with these fats is not recommended.*

which to ditch

SATURATED

Man-made fats are never healthy. Trans fats are particularly harmful.

"Buttery spreads," including oil blends like Earth Balance, Benecol, and I Can't Believe It's Not Butter

Hydrogenated or partially hydrogenated oils

Margarine

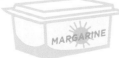

UNSATURATED

These oils are highly processed and oxidize easily via one or more of the following: light, air, or heat. Consuming oxidized oils is never healthy.

Canola oil (rapeseed oil)

Corn oil

Grapeseed oil

Rice bran oil

Safflower oil

Soybean oil

Sunflower oil

Vegetable oil

For more detailed information on the fatty acid profiles of fats & oils, check out my book Practical Paleo.

CHOOSING COOKING FATS

listed in order of most stable to least stable for cooking

The fats and oils are ranked below based on the following criteria: (1) how they're made—choose naturally occurring, minimally processed options first; (2) their fatty acid composition—the more saturated they are, the more stable and less likely to be damaged or oxidized they are; (3) smoke point—this tells you how hot is too hot before you will damage the fats, though it should be considered a secondary factor to fatty acid profile.

VERY STABLE
—IDEAL FOR COOKING

Butter/ghee

Cocoa butter

Coconut oil

Duck fat

Lard/bacon fat (pork fat)

Palm oil from sustainable sources

Tallow/suet (beef fat)

MODERATELY STABLE
—BEST COLD

Avocado oil*

Macadamia nut oil*

Olive oil*

Rice bran oil*

LEAST STABLE
—NOT RECOMMENDED

Canola oil**

Corn oil**

Grapeseed oil**

Safflower oil**

Sesame seed oil**

Soybean oil**

Sunflower oil**

Vegetable shortening**

Walnut oil*

* While not recommended for cooking, cold-pressed nut and seed oils that are stored in the refrigerator may be used to finish recipes or after cooking is completed, for flavor.

** These oils are not recommended for consumption, whether hot or cold, but are listed here for your reference, as they are commonly used.

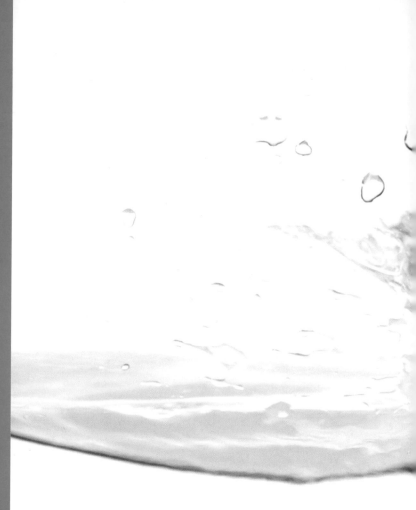

MEAL
PLANS
& RECIPES

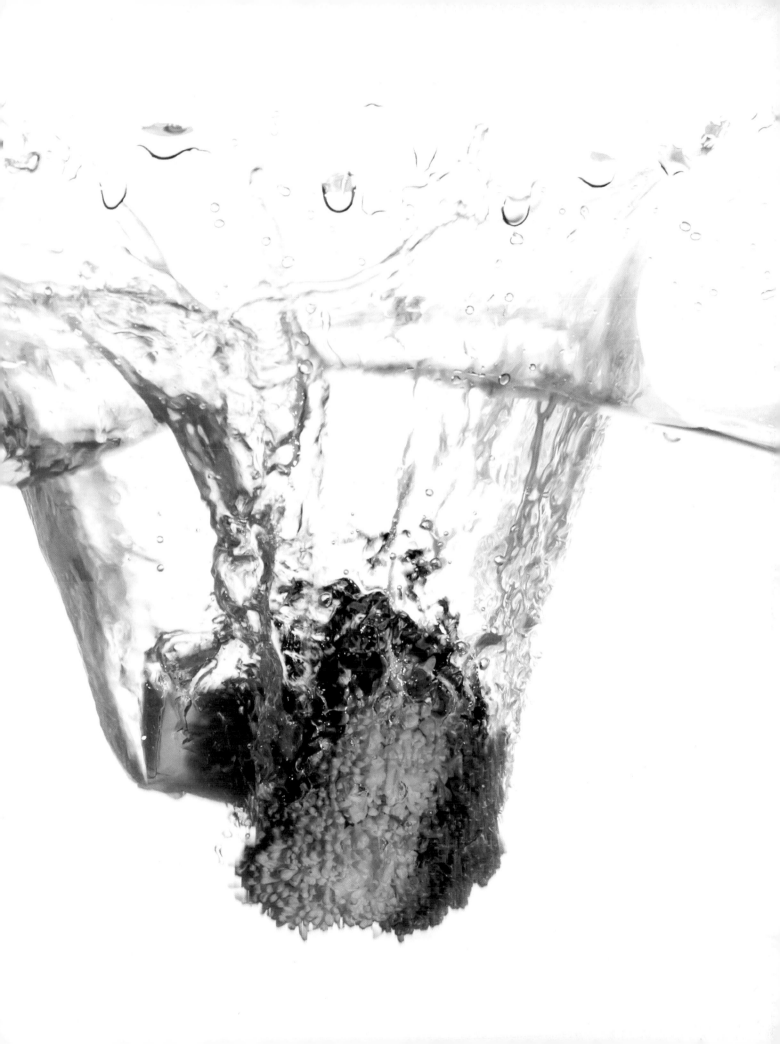

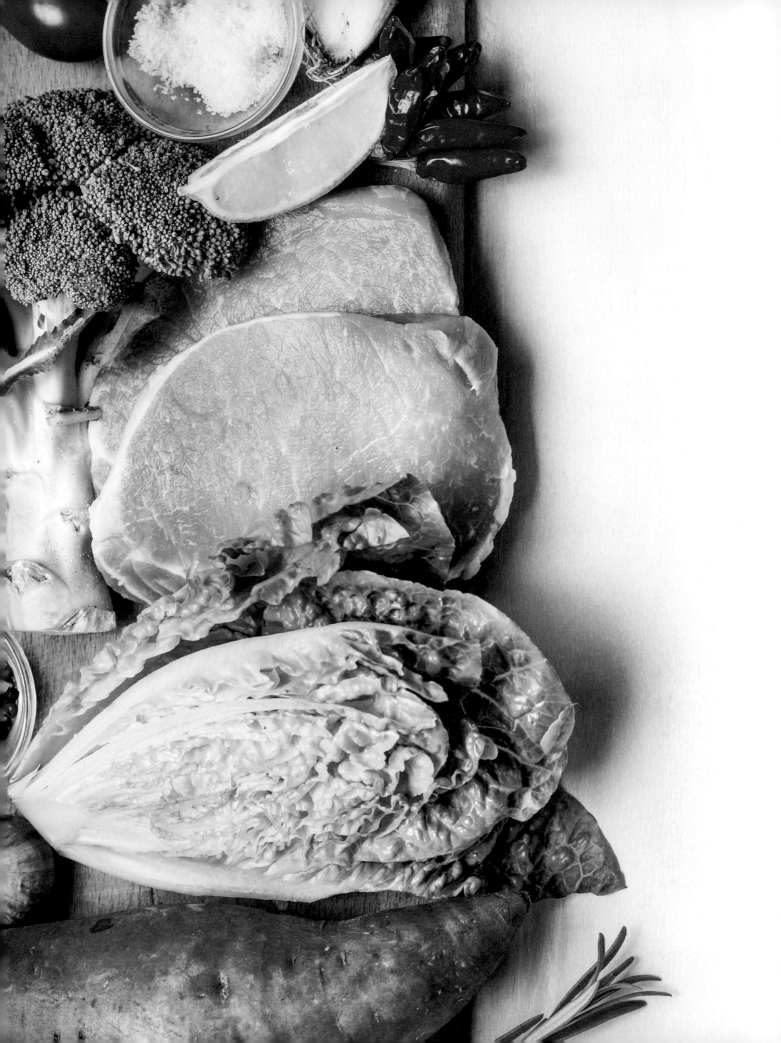

THE 21-DAY SUGAR DETOX
MEAL PLAN

Upon first glance, this meal plan might look a little intense, but it's actually quite simple to follow, and I'm going to be with you every step of the way.

While you'll need to do some cooking (this is a real-food detox, after all!), I designed this plan so that your time in the kitchen will be more productive and you won't have to cook every day.

This plan mimics how I typically cook and will help you become more comfortable in the kitchen long-term. Leftovers are anything but dull in my mind, and I love to get creative in making recipes work together easily, without compromising flavor.

Here's what you'll find in the following pages:

PREP
This includes grocery shopping and defrosting meat.

BREAKFAST / LUNCH / DINNER / SNACK
This is where you can find what you'll eat each day.

MAKE AHEAD
In this section, I break down the recipes or components that you'll be making that day to eat later.

SAVE
Aka leftovers. You can quickly glance at this row to see what food you'll have left over from the day's meals and when you'll be eating it later on.

COOKING DAY vs EASY COOKING DAY
Cooking days are more intense: you'll be prepping multiple recipes for later as well as making the meals for that day. Easy cooking days involve some minor cooking, but the prep is minimal and I've made sure the recipes are simple and easy to follow.

Weekly shopping lists for this plan are on pages 122 to 124. Before you head to the store, check your fridge and pantry to see what items you already have on hand.

Keep in mind that the plan is designed for one person and the recipes generally make enough for two servings, so there will be leftovers—which are used later in the plan! If you're cooking for more than one person, adjust the portions accordingly.

For recipes that contain 21DSD fruit, factor this into your total intake of allowed fruit for the day.

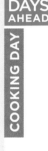

TWO DAYS AHEAD — COOKING DAY

PREP
- Grocery shopping (freeze any meat that you won't use within 2 days)

MAKE AHEAD
- *Soak 1 cup cashews for tomorrow's "cheese" sauce (Level 3 or dairy-free)
- *Bake 1 small sweet potato for tomorrow's "cheese" sauce (Level 3 or dairy-free)
- Bake 2 small sweet potatoes for dinner day 1
- Make all spice blends (pages 248–249)
- Make 2 servings Smoky Toasted Nut Mix (page 212)

ONE DAY AHEAD — COOKING DAY

DINNER

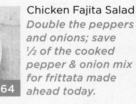

Chicken Fajita Salad
Double the peppers and onions; save ½ of the cooked pepper & onion mix for frittata made ahead today.

164

MAKE AHEAD
- **Make mayonnaise (page 246)
- Make Banana Nut Smoothie (page 142) for breakfast days 2 & 5
- Hard-boil 4 eggs for breakfast days 2 & 5
- Make 2 batches Ranch Dressing (page 240)
- *Make Cashew "Cheese" Sauce (page 235) for dinner day 6 (Level 3 or dairy-free)
- *Make Peanut Sauce (page 234) for breakfast days 4, 10 & 13
- Make 21DSD Frozen Coco-Monkey Bites (page 222) for snacks
- Make salad dressing of choice (pages 238–240) for dinner day 3 & lunch day 5
- Cook 2 chicken breasts for lunch days 2 & 4
- Make Sausage, Spinach & Peppers Frittata (page 138) for breakfast days 1 & 3

SAVE
- 1 serving dinner salad for day 1 lunch
- ½ avocado for day 1 snack

* optional   ** or purchase

DAY 1 — COOKING DAY

BREAKFAST

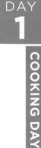

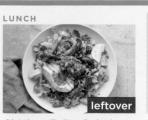
138
Sausage, Spinach & Peppers Frittata

LUNCH

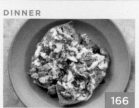
leftover
Chicken Fajita Salad

DINNER

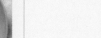
166
Ranch Chicken & Bacon Stuffed Potatoes

SNACK

1/2 avocado + salsa with raw veggies

MAKE AHEAD
• Make Smoky Chicken Salad Lettuce Boats (page 172) for lunch day 2 using breasts cooked day before detox
• Cook 4 slices bacon for lunch days 3 & 6

SAVE
• 1 serving frittata for breakfast day 3
• 1 serving stuffed potato for dinner day 2

DAY 2

BREAKFAST

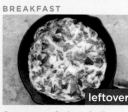
142
½ Banana Nut Smoothie + 2 hard-boiled eggs

LUNCH

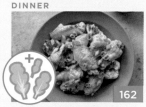
172
Smoky Chicken Salad Lettuce Boats
(assemble in a.m.)

DINNER

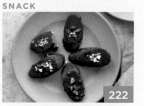
leftover
Ranch Chicken & Bacon Stuffed Potatoes

SNACK

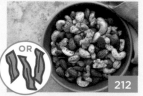
212
Smoky Toasted Nut Mix or jerky

notes _____
_____
_____

DAY 3 — EASY COOKING DAY

BREAKFAST

leftover
Sausage, Spinach & Peppers Frittata

LUNCH

On each of 2 leaves lettuce, layer 2 slices bacon, 1–2 slices turkey, tomato slices, avocado slices, mayo & mustard

DINNER

162
Buffalo Cauliflower & Chicken Wings + green salad

SNACK

222
21DSD Frozen Coco-Monkey Bites

SAVE
• 1 serving wings + salad for lunch day 5

DAY 4 — COOKING DAY

BREAKFAST

130
Breakfast Salad

LUNCH

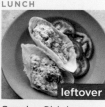
leftover
Smoky Chicken Salad Lettuce Boats
(assemble in a.m.)

DINNER

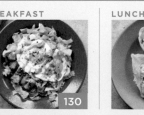
194
Crispy Brussels Sprouts

Season 4 oz. steak with spice blend of choice & grill to desired doneness (see page 168)

SNACK

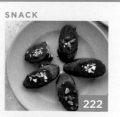
222
21DSD Frozen Coco-Monkey Bites

MAKE AHEAD
• Bake 2 small sweet potatoes for dinner day 6 and lunch day 8 (bake with Brussels sprouts)
• Make Bacon, Brussels, Asparagus & Goat Cheese Frittata (page 140) for breakfast days 6 & 7

BREAKFAST

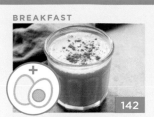

142

½ Banana Nut Smoothie
+ 2 hard-boiled eggs

LUNCH

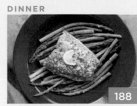

leftover

Buffalo Cauliflower &
Chicken Wings
+ green salad

DINNER

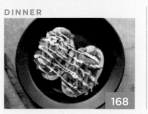

188

½ *batch* Super Garlic
Salmon & Vegetables
*(leave half salmon and
half vegetables uncooked
for lunch day 7)*

SNACK

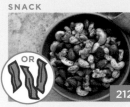

212

Smoky Toasted Nut Mix
or jerky

SAVE

- 1 serving salmon & vegetables (uncooked) for
lunch day 7

BREAKFAST

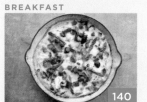

140

- Bacon, Brussels,
Asparagus & Goat Cheese
Frittata

LUNCH

*On each of 2 leaves
lettuce, layer 2 slices
bacon, 1–2 slices turkey,
tomato slices, avocado
slices, mayo & mustard*

DINNER

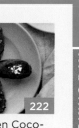

168

Cheesesteak Stuffed Potatoes
using baked potatoes from day 4

SNACK

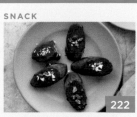

222

21DSD Frozen Coco-
Monkey Bites

PREP

- Grocery shopping (freeze
any meat that you won't
use within 2 days)

MAKE AHEAD

- Make 21DSD
Ketchup (page
232)

- Make Smoky Toasted
Nut Mix (page 212)
for snacks

SAVE

- 1 serving frittata
for breakfast
day 7

- 1 serving
stuffed potato
for lunch day 8

BREAKFAST

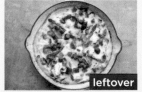

leftover

Bacon, Brussels,
Asparagus & Goat
Cheese Frittata

LUNCH

188

½ *batch* Super Garlic
Salmon & Vegetables
*(use remaining ingredients
from dinner day 5)*

DINNER

176

Tangy Chicken Salad

SNACK

222

21DSD Frozen Coco-
Monkey Bites

MAKE AHEAD

- Make Pumpkin Spice Smoothie (page 145) for
breakfast days 8, 9 & 11

- Hard-boil 6 eggs for breakfast days 8, 9 & 11

- **Make Healthy Homemade Mayonnaise (page 246)

- Make Ranch Dressing (page 240)

- Make 21DSD BBQ Sauce (page 233)

- Make 21DSD Cinnamon Banana Bread (page 220) for
snacks

SAVE

- 1 serving chicken salad for lunch day 9

notes _____

_____

_____

_____

_____

_____

* optional   ** or purchase

*This meal plan is designed for 1 person, so recipes that make 2 servings yield leftovers.
If you're cooking for more than 1 person, increase portions accordingly.*

DAY 8
EASY COOKING DAY

BREAKFAST
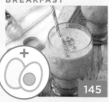
145
⅓ Pumpkin Spice Smoothie + 2 hard-boiled eggs

LUNCH
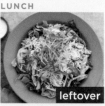
leftover
Cheesesteak Stuffed Potatoes

DINNER
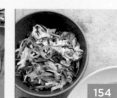
182
Grilled Pork Fall Salad

SNACK
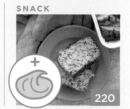
OR
212
Smoky Toasted Nut Mix or jerky

SAVE
• 1 serving pork salad for lunch day 11

notes _____
_____
_____

DAY 9
COOKING DAY

BREAKFAST
145
⅓ Pumpkin Spice Smoothie + 2 hard-boiled eggs

LUNCH
leftover
Tangy Chicken Salad

DINNER
154
BBQ Burger
154
Spicy Slaw
double batch

SNACK
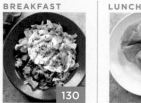
220
2 slices banana bread + nut butter

MAKE AHEAD
• Make Slow Cooker BBQ Pulled Pork (page 158) for dinner days 10, 17 & 19

SAVE
• 1 serving burger + slaw for lunch day 10

DAY 10

BREAKFAST
130
Breakfast Salad

LUNCH
leftover
BBQ Burger
leftover
Spicy Slaw

DINNER
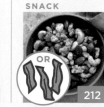
158
leftover
BBQ Pulled Pork Tacos with Spicy Slaw

SNACK
OR
212
Smoky Toasted Nut Mix or jerky

PREP
• Freeze ½ batch slow cooker pork (a.m.)

SAVE
• 1 serving tacos for lunch day 12

notes _____
_____
_____

DAY 11
EASY COOKING DAY

BREAKFAST
145
⅓ Pumpkin Spice Smoothie + 2 hard-boiled eggs

LUNCH
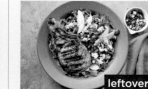
leftover
Grilled Pork Fall Salad

DINNER
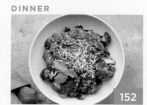
152
B3 Bowl
Make a double batch of Crispy Broccoli and use in frittata made ahead today

SNACK
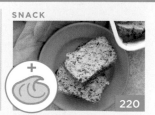
220
2 slices banana bread + nut butter

MAKE AHEAD
• Make Broccoli, Ham & Cheese Frittata (page 136) for breakfast days 12 & 14

SAVE
• 1 serving B3 Bowl for dinner day 13

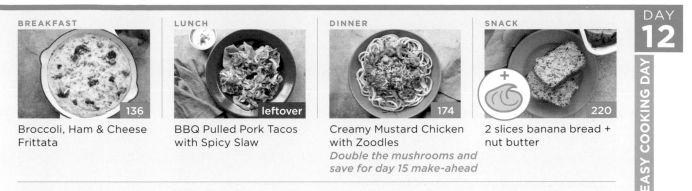

BREAKFAST	LUNCH	DINNER	SNACK
136	leftover	174	220
Broccoli, Ham & Cheese Frittata	BBQ Pulled Pork Tacos with Spicy Slaw	Creamy Mustard Chicken with Zoodles *Double the mushrooms and save for day 15 make-ahead*	2 slices banana bread + nut butter

SAVE
- 1 lb sliced cooked mushrooms for make-ahead day 15
- 1 serving chicken for lunch day 13

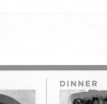

BREAKFAST	LUNCH	DINNER	SNACK
130	leftover	leftover	212
Breakfast Salad	Creamy Mustard Chicken with Zoodles	B3 Bowl	Smoky Toasted Nut Mix or jerky

PREP
- Grocery shopping

notes _____

_____

_____

BREAKFAST	LUNCH	DINNER			SNACK
leftover	178	170	198	206	220
Broccoli, Ham & Cheese Frittata	Deli Tuna Sliders	Diane's Simple Roast Chicken	Pesto Roasted Carrots	Ranch Roasted Potatoes	2 slices banana bread + nut butter

MAKE AHEAD
- Make Apple Pie Smoothie (page 144) for breakfast days 15, 18 & 20
- Hard-boil 6 eggs for breakfast days 15, 18 & 20
- **Make Healthy Homemade Mayonnaise (page 246)
- Make 2 batches Ranch Dressing (page 240)
- *Make Peanut Sauce (page 234) for breakfast day 21
- Make Two-Bite Chocolate Cream Pies (page 218) for snacks
- Make Smoky Toasted Nut Mix (page 212) for snacks

SAVE
- 1 serving tuna for lunch day 16
- 1 serving Pesto Roasted Carrots for lunch day 15
- Remaining pesto for lunch day 15 and breakfast days 16 & 17
- 1 serving roast chicken for lunch day 15
- 2 servings roast chicken for make-ahead day 15
- 1 serving roasted potatoes for lunch day 15
- 2 servings roasted potatoes for breakfast days 16 & 17

* *optional*   ** *or purchase*

This meal plan is designed for 1 person, so recipes that make 2 servings yield leftovers. If you're cooking for more than 1 person, increase portions accordingly.

BREAKFAST

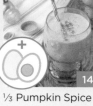

145

⅓ Pumpkin Spice Smoothie + 2 hard-boiled eggs

LUNCH

Assemble a Buddha bowl from the leftover roast chicken, pesto, carrots & potatoes (or zoodles if leftover from lunch day 13)

DINNER

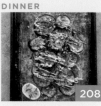

208

Roasted Eggplant Steaks with Tahini Sauce

Season 4 oz. steak with spice blend of choice & grill to desired doneness (see page 168)

SNACK

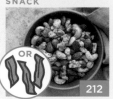

212

Smoky Toasted Nut Mix or jerky

MAKE AHEAD
- Make Roasted Butternut Squash (page 202) for lunch days 17 & 19
- Make Mushroom, Pesto & Goat Cheese Frittata (page 134) for breakfast day 16: add roast chicken from day 14 and use mushrooms from day 12

SAVE
- 1 serving eggplant steaks for dinner day 16

notes _____
_____
_____
_____
_____

BREAKFAST

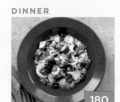 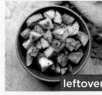

134   leftover

Mushroom, Pesto & Goat Cheese Frittata   Ranch Roasted Potatoes

LUNCH

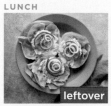

leftover

Deli Tuna Sliders

DINNER

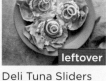

180

Mediterranean Meatball Bowl

SNACK

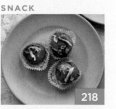

218

Two-Bite Chocolate Cream Pies

PREP
- Defrost slow cooker pork before 5 p.m.

MAKE AHEAD
- Roast 1 head garlic for dinner day 18
- Cook chicken thighs for lunch days 17 & 19

SAVE
- 1 serving Mediterranean Meatball Bowl for lunch day 18

BREAKFAST

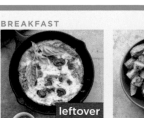

leftover   leftover

Mushroom, Pesto & Goat Cheese Frittata   Ranch Roasted Potatoes

LUNCH

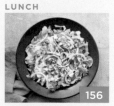

156

BBQ Chicken Salad

DINNER

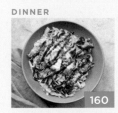

160

BBQ Pulled Pork Buddha Bowl

SNACK

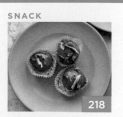

218

Two-Bite Chocolate Cream Pies

SAVE
- 1 serving BBQ Pulled Pork Buddha Bowl for dinner day 19
- 1 serving BBQ Chicken Salad for lunch day 19

notes _____
_____
_____

DAY 18

BREAKFAST

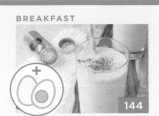

144

⅓ Apple Pie Smoothie +
2 hard-boiled eggs

LUNCH

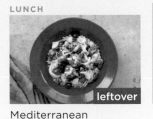

leftover

Mediterranean
Meatball Bowl

DINNER

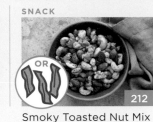

186

Sausage & Spinach
"Polenta" Bowl

SNACK

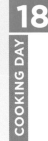

OR

212

Smoky Toasted Nut Mix
or jerky

MAKE AHEAD
- Make Sausage, Spinach & Peppers Frittata (page 138) for breakfast day 19 & lunch day 20

SAVE
- 1 serving polenta bowl for lunch day 21

DAY 19

BREAKFAST

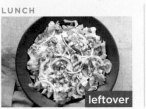

138

Sausage, Spinach
& Peppers Frittata

LUNCH

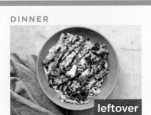

leftover

BBQ Chicken Salad

DINNER

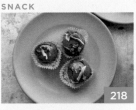

leftover

BBQ Pulled Pork
Buddha Bowl

SNACK

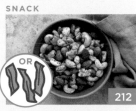

218

Two-Bite Chocolate
Cream Pies

SAVE
- 1 serving frittata for lunch day 20

notes _____
_____
_____

DAY 20

BREAKFAST

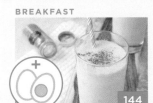

144

⅓ Apple Pie Smoothie +
2 hard-boiled eggs

LUNCH

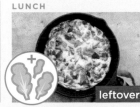

leftover

Sausage, Spinach &
Peppers Frittata +
green salad

DINNER

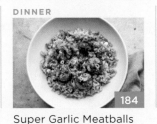

184

Super Garlic Meatballs
with Fried Rice

SNACK

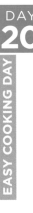

212

Smoky Toasted Nut Mix
or jerky

SAVE
- 1 serving garlic meatballs for dinner day 21

notes _____
_____

DAY 21

BREAKFAST

130

Breakfast Salad

LUNCH

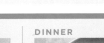

leftover

Sausage & Spinach
"Polenta" Bowl

DINNER

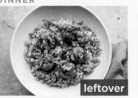

leftover

Super Garlic Meatballs
with Fried Rice

SNACK

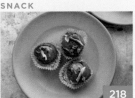

218

Two-Bite Chocolate
Cream Pies

*optional   ** or purchase*

*This meal plan is designed for 1 person, so recipes that make 2 servings yield leftovers.
If you're cooking for more than 1 person, increase portions accordingly.*

Week 1 Shopping List

PRODUCE

asparagus, 1 pound (about 1 bunch), or green beans, 1 pound

asparagus, ⅛ pound (½ cup chopped)

avocados, 2

bananas, green-tipped, 8 medium

basil leaves, about ¼ bunch (¼ cup chopped)

broccoli, 1 large head

Brussels sprouts, 1 pound

cauliflower, 2 medium to large heads

celery, about ½ stalk

chives, fresh, 2 tablespoons chopped

cilantro, fresh, ¼ cup chopped

fennel, about ⅛ pound (½ cup sliced)

garlic, 4 cloves

green apples, 2

green bell pepper, 1

green onion, 1 (2 tablespoons chopped)

kale, about ⅓ pound (2 cups chopped)

lemons, 4 medium

lime, ½

onions (yellow, red, or a combination), 4 small

potatoes, white or sweet, 2 large

red bell peppers, 2

red onions, 3 small + 2 medium

romaine lettuce, 1½ pounds

ruby red grapefruit, 1

spinach, ¼ pound

sweet potatoes, 2 large

tomatoes, 2

yellow bell peppers, 2

yellow onions, 2 small

FOR SERVING

carrots

celery

green salad

MEAT & SEAFOOD

bacon, 1 pound

chicken breasts, 2 pounds

chicken thighs, bone-in, with skin, 2 pounds

chicken wings, 2 pounds

deli turkey, 4 to 8 slices

ground pork, ½ pound

precooked 21DSD-approved breakfast sausages, 1 or 2

skirt steak, flank steak, or chicken breast, 1 pound

steak, 4 ounces (¼ pound)

wild salmon, 2 (6-ounce) fillets

SEASONINGS, OILS, AND BAKING INGREDIENTS

allspice, ¼ teaspoon

apple cider vinegar, ¼ cup + 3 tablespoons

baking soda, 1½ teaspoons

carob powder, unsweetened, 2 tablespoons

cashew flour, 1 cup

celery powder, ½ tablespoon

chili powder, ¼ cup + ½ tablespoon

chipotle powder, 1 tablespoon + 1 teaspoon

cocoa powder, unsweetened, 2 tablespoons

coconut aminos, ½ cup

coconut flour, ¾ cup

coconut oil, ¼ cup + 3 tablespoons

dill weed, 2½ tablespoons

dried chives, 5 tablespoons

dried garlic flakes, 1¼ cups

dried ground sage, 1 tablespoon

dried lemon peel, 2 tablespoons + 2½ teaspoons

dried onion flakes, 5 tablespoons

dried oregano leaves, 3 tablespoons + 1 teaspoon

dried parsley, ¼ cup + 1½ tablespoons

extra-virgin olive oil, ¾ cup + 2 tablespoons

fennel seeds, 1 tablespoon

fish sauce, 2 to 3 dashes

garlic powder, 3 tablespoons + ½ teaspoon

ginger powder, ¼ teaspoon

granulated garlic, ½ cup + ½ tablespoon

granulated onion, ¼ cup + ½ tablespoon

ground cinnamon, 2 tablespoons + 2 teaspoons

ground cloves, 2 pinches

mustard powder, 3½ teaspoons

onion powder, 3 tablespoons

paprika, ½ cup + 1 tablespoon + ½ teaspoon

poppy seeds, 3⅓ tablespoons

pumpkin pie spice, 1 teaspoon

pure vanilla extract, 2¾ teaspoons

red pepper flakes, ¼ teaspoon

red wine vinegar, ¼ cup

rice vinegar, ¼ cup

sesame seeds, 3 tablespoons + ½ teaspoon

smoked paprika, 2 tablespoons

sweet paprika, 1 tablespoon

vanilla bean pod, ¼, or pure vanilla extract, ½ teaspoon

PANTRY ITEMS

almond butter, ¼ cup

canned pumpkin, ¼ cup

coconut cream, 2¼ cups (or three 13½-ounce cans of full-fat coconut milk)

hot sauce, sugar-free/sweetener-free, 3 tablespoons

mayonnaise, 2 tablespoons (or homemade, page 246)

nuts, raw, 2 cups

peanut butter or other nut or seed butter, ½ cup + 2 tablespoons

tomato paste, 6 ounces

CHEESE (Levels 1 & 2 only)

goat cheese, 2 ounces

mizithra, feta cheese, or goat cheese, full-fat, 4 ounces

EGGS AND NUT MILKS

almond milk or cashew milk, full-fat, 1 cup (or homemade, page 242)

coconut milk, full-fat, 2 cups + 3 tablespoons (or homemade, page 243)

eggs, 2 dozen

MISC.

cooking fat, ¼ cup + 1 tablespoon + 2 teaspoons

ghee, ¼ cup + 2 tablespoons

pico de gallo, 2 tablespoons

salsa, for serving

If making Healthy Homemade Mayonnaise (page 246)

Dijon mustard, gluten-free, 2 teaspoons

eggs, 4

extra-virgin olive oil, ½ cup

lemon juice, 2 tablespoons

macadamia nut oil or other oil, 1 cup

If making Cashew "Cheese" Sauce (page 235)

cashews, raw, 1 cup

garlic powder, 1 teaspoon

nutritional yeast, 1 cup

onion powder, 1 teaspoon

paprika, ½ teaspoon

sweet potato, about ¼ pound

Week 2 Shopping List

PRODUCE

arugula, ½ pound

avocado, 1

banana, green-tipped, 1 medium

basil leaves, 2 bunches (2 cups tightly packed)

broccoli, 2 large heads

butter lettuce, 10 leaves

carrots, 9 medium

celery, about ½ stalk

cilantro, ¼ cup chopped

coleslaw mix, 2 (16-ounce) bags (or an equivalent amount of shredded cabbage and carrots)

garlic, 15 to 17 cloves (about 1½ heads)

green apples, 2

jalapeño peppers, 2

lemons, 1½ medium

mushrooms (sliced), 2 pounds

red onions, 2 small + 2 medium

romaine lettuce, ¼ pound (1 cup chopped)

romaine lettuce leaves, 6 large, or butter lettuce leaves, 10 small

shallot or garlic, ½ teaspoon minced

tomato, 1 medium

yellow onions, 2 medium

yellow or red potatoes, 1 pound

zucchini, 2 large or 4 small

MEAT & SEAFOOD

chicken, 1 whole (about 3½ to 4 pounds)

chicken thighs, 1 pound boneless, skinless, or 2 pounds bone-in

ground beef, 1 pound

ground pork, ½ pound

ham, cooked, ½ pound

pork chops, bone-in, 2 (1 inch thick; 6 to 8 ounces each)

pork shoulder roast, 4 pounds

precooked 21DSD-approved breakfast sausages, 1 or 2

SEASONINGS, OILS, AND BAKING INGREDIENTS

apple cider vinegar, ½ teaspoon

balsamic vinegar, ⅓ cup

carob powder, unsweetened, 1 tablespoon

cocoa powder, unsweetened, 2 tablespoons

coconut aminos, ½ cup

dried ground oregano, 2 teaspoons

extra-virgin olive oil, 1¾ cups

fish sauce, 2 to 3 dashes

garlic powder, 1¼ teaspoons

ground cinnamon, 2 teaspoons

nutmeg, 2 dashes

onion powder, 1½ teaspoons

pure vanilla extract, 1¼ teaspoons

red pepper flakes, ½ teaspoon

red wine vinegar, ¼ cup + 2 tablespoons

rice vinegar, ¼ cup

sesame seeds , ½ teaspoon

PANTRY ITEMS

almond butter, 2 tablespoons

almonds, raw, 1 cup

cashews or walnuts, raw, ½ cup chopped

chicken broth, 1½ cups (or homemade, page 244)

coconut, unsweetened finely shredded, ½ cup

coconut cream, ¾ cup (or one 13½-ounce can of full-fat coconut milk)

Dijon mustard, gluten-free, 1 tablespoon + 1 teaspoon

mayonnaise, 4 to 6 tablespoons (or homemade, page 246)

nuts, raw, 1 cup

pasta sauce, sugar-free, 1 (24-ounce) jar

peanut butter or other nut or seed butter, ½ cup

pine nuts, ¼ cup, or walnut halves, ½ cup

tuna, 2 (6-ounce) cans

CHEESE *(Levels 1 & 2 only)*

blue cheese or goat cheese, 2 tablespoons crumbled

cheddar cheese, 4 ounces

grated cheese of choice, for topping

hard cheese, such as Parmigiano-Reggiano or Pecorino Romano, 1 ounce (¼ cup shredded)

EGGS AND NUT MILKS

coconut milk, full-fat, 2 cups (or homemade, page 243)

eggs, 7

MISC.

cooking fat, ¾ cup + 2 tablespoons

ghee, 1 tablespoon

If making Healthy Homemade Mayonnaise (page 246)

Dijon mustard, gluten-free, 1 teaspoon

eggs, 2

extra-virgin olive oil, ¼ cup

lemon, 1 small

macadamia nut oil or other oil, ½ cup

Week 3 Shopping List

PRODUCE

basil leaves, about ¼ bunch (¼ cup + 1 tablespoon chopped)

butternut squash, 1 large (2 to 3 pounds)

cauliflower, 2 large heads

cilantro, 1 bunch (1¼ cups chopped)

cilantro, basil, or mint (or any combination), ½ cup chopped

cucumber, 1 medium

eggplant, 1 large

garlic, 1 head + 12 cloves (about 2 heads)

green onions, 1 bunch (1 cup chopped)

lemons, 4 medium

red bell peppers, 2

red onions, 1 medium + 1½ small

romaine hearts, 2

romaine lettuce, ¼ pound

spinach, 1 pound

tomato, 1

yellow bell pepper, 1

yellow onion, 1 medium

FOR SERVING

green salad

MEAT & SEAFOOD

chicken thighs, bone-in, with skin, 2 pounds

ground lamb or beef, 1 pound

ground pork or other higher-fat ground meat, 1 pound

ground pork, 2 pounds

precooked 21DSD-approved breakfast sausages, 1 or 2

steak, 4 ounces (¼ pound)

SEASONINGS, OILS, AND BAKING INGREDIENTS

apple cider vinegar, 1 teaspoon

coconut aminos, 1 cup

dried ground oregano, 1 teaspoon

extra-virgin olive oil, ¾ cup + 2 tablespoons

fish sauce, ½ teaspoon

garlic powder, 1 teaspoon

ginger powder, ½ teaspoon

granulated garlic, ½ teaspoon

granulated onion, ¼ teaspoon

paprika, ¼ teaspoon

sesame oil, 2 teaspoons

PANTRY ITEMS

almonds, raw, 1 cup

coconut cream, 1½ cups (or two 13½-ounce cans of full-fat coconut milk)

diced tomatoes, 1 (28-ounce) can

Kalamata olives, whole or sliced, ¼ cup

pine nuts, toasted, 2 tablespoons

tahini, ½ cup

CHEESE (Levels 1 & 2 only)

goat cheese, 2 ounces

Parmesan cheese, ½ cup grated

EGGS AND NUT MILKS

coconut milk, full-fat, ¼ cup (or homemade, page 243)

eggs, 10 or 11

MISC.

cooking fat, ¾ cup + 1 tablespoon

riced cauliflower, 3 (12-ounce) packages

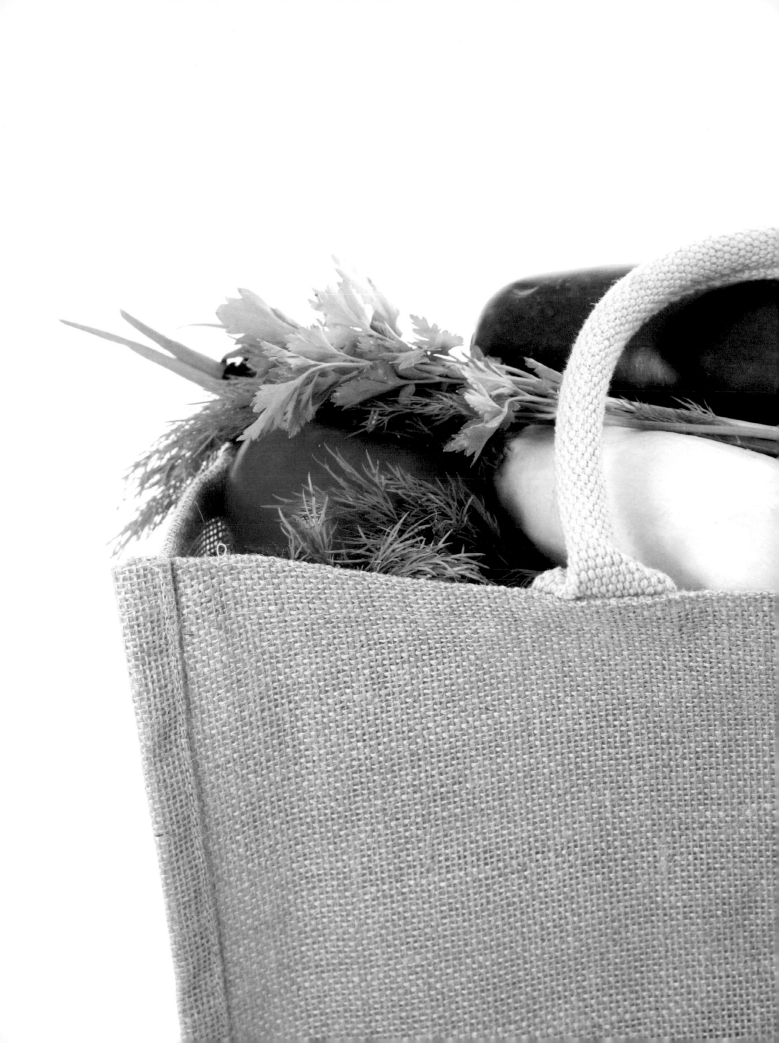

Notes on the Recipes and Ingredients

The recipes in this book are primarily intended to be used with the meal plan on pages 115 to 121, but you are welcome to build your own meal plan from these recipes or from recipes in *The 21-Day Sugar Detox* or *The 21-Day Sugar Detox Cookbook* as well.

Some ingredients in the recipes may be new to you or can be a little bit confusing. The following notes will help clarify what to use and how to select ingredients.

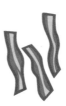

BACON, SAUSAGE & CURED MEATS

I know this one can be extremely confusing, but it's one of the few exceptions to the no-added-sugar-or-sweeteners rule on the 21DSD. When sugar is used in curing meats, it's generally a trace amount, and little to no sugar remains in the finished food. So, look for bacon, sausage, and cured meats with less than 1 gram of sugar on the Nutrition Facts label (which will be indicated as "0 grams" even when sugar is in the ingredients list). Sausage may not include any of the fruits on the No list (page 21). While many premade sausage varieties include apples, they are not likely green or Granny Smith apples, and I recommend avoiding them. If you'd like to have sausage that includes apples, you can make delicious breakfast sausage patties by adding 2 tablespoons of Italian Spice Blend (page 248) and ½ of a diced green apple to any ground meat.

COOKING FAT

When a recipe calls for simply "cooking fat," you may choose any cooking fat featured in the Guide to Healthy Fats & Oils (page 111). I generally recommend either ghee or coconut oil as a primary cooking fat. Olive oil may also be used over low to medium heat, but take care not to allow it to burn or smoke in your pan before use.

COCONUT AMINOS

This is a soy-free and gluten-free replacement for traditional soy sauce. Coconut Secret and Trader Joe's brand tend to be sweeter than soy sauce, while Big Tree brand is pretty similar to the original. I recommend tasting the product before using it in your recipe to see if it seems strong or slightly sweet, and adjusting how much you use accordingly. In sauces that are reduced, I recommend using the sweeter coconut aminos, whereas in a stir fry or fried rice recipe, I recommend using the stronger, more traditional-tasting version. Note that these products will list "coconut sap" or "coconut nectar" as an ingredient but are completely approved for the 21DSD because they are fermented.

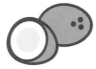

COCONUT CREAM & COCONUT MILK

You can buy coconut cream or you can get it from coconut milk. To get the "cream" from a 13½-ounce can of full-fat coconut milk, chill it for at least eight hours, then open the can and scoop out the thick cream on the top.

In recipes, I generally recommend full-fat coconut milk, though you may choose to use a lite version for smoothies. You may also use almond milk, cashew milk, or any other nut milk, or even full-fat (whole) regular milk on Levels 1 and 2. I highly recommend using grass-fed milk if you're using dairy.

CAROB POWDER

A caffeine-free and less-bitter replacement for cacao powder, carob powder adds a hint of sweetness without any sweetener, so it's worth buying if you can find it! (While caffeine isn't limited or restricted on the 21DSD, many find that they are sensitive to it.) If you can't find carob powder, you may use cocoa powder in its place.

CHEESE (dairy)

If you are following Level 1 or 2 of the 21DSD, you may use full-fat cheese as you wish in recipes or as a snack. I recommend organic and/or grass-fed varieties whenever possible. Remember that portion sizes matter, but you need to determine what's best for you using the guide on pages 22 and 23.

NUTRITIONAL YEAST

This is a slightly cheesy-flavored *deactivated* yeast (it will not work in baking recipes to leaven anything) to use in place of a grated cheese topping or in recipes when avoiding dairy (this applies to anyone on Level 3 of the 21DSD as well as anyone who wishes to avoid dairy). Nutritional yeast contains B-complex vitamins and can be found either in bulk or with other dairy-free items at the grocery store. I recommend keeping it refrigerated once opened, though this isn't required. One popular, widely available brand of nutritional yeast is Bragg's.

HOT SAUCE

When looking for a 21DSD-friendly hot sauce, check ingredient labels for any forms of added sugar or gluten (malt vinegars or hydrolyzed proteins). While an organic hot sauce is ideal, a favorite in many recipes is Frank's Red Hot for its classic Buffalo-style flavor. Other brands of hot sauces that are free of sugar or sweeteners are Tabasco and Arizona Gunslinger/Arizona Pepper's Organic Harvest Foods. Always read labels, though, as ingredients may change over time!

RICED CAULIFLOWER

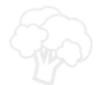

If a recipe calls for riced cauliflower, you can make it from a large head of raw cauliflower by pulsing coarsely chopped florets in a food processor until the texture is crumbly, or you can buy a package of riced cauliflower. Riced cauliflower is readily available both frozen and fresh at most grocery stores. Frozen will last longer, but fresh may cook slightly faster. When making cauliflower mash or polenta, it's best to use a fresh head of cauliflower because pre-riced cauliflower may be too dry to yield a smooth result.

SEA SALT AND GROUND BLACK PEPPER

In general, this refers to finely ground versions of both, though you may choose to finish a dish with some additional coarse or Maldon sea salt or freshly cracked black pepper. Always season as you cook, and taste your food (when the meat is no longer raw or, with a veggie-based dish, while cooking) to ensure you won't need to add much salt and/or pepper at the table. This will yield more flavorful food without making it salty or overly peppery.

"Season lightly" means to use a few pinches, while "season generously" or "season liberally" means to evenly coat the surface of whatever you are cooking (typically meat, potatoes, or other raw items that can handle a hearty amount of seasoning). Don't be shy with seasonings; doing so will result in bland food.

TOMATO SAUCE (PASTA SAUCE/MARINARA)

When looking for a 21DSD-friendly tomato sauce, check ingredient labels for any forms of added sugar and vegetable oils like soybean or canola oil. While an organic tomato sauce is ideal, one with "clean" ingredients is perfectly okay! Some brands I love, if you aren't making your own, are Yellow Barn Organic/Biodynamic and RAO's (not organic). Always continue to read all labels, though, as ingredients may change over time!

BREAK-FAST

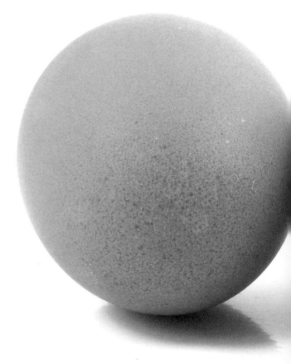

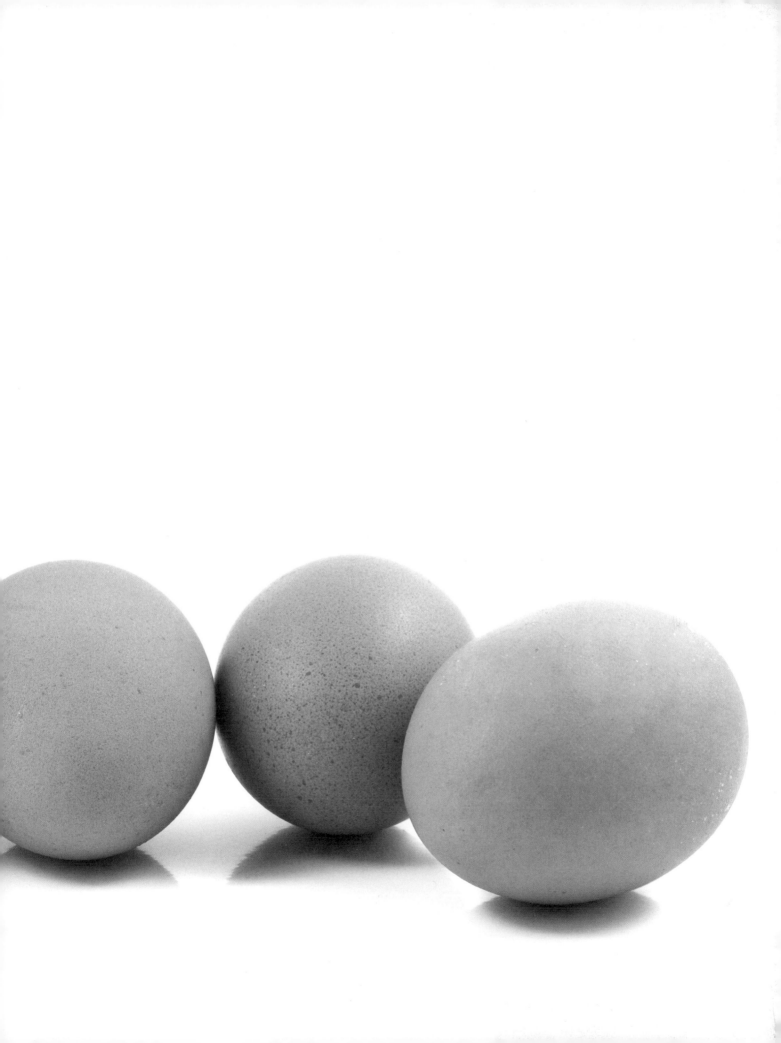

Breakfast Salad

PREP TIME **5 MINUTES** • COOK TIME **5 MINUTES** • MAKES **1 SERVING**

NUTS
EGGS
NIGHTSHADES
FODMAPS

2 to 3 teaspoons cooking fat, plus more for the egg

2 or 3 eggs

1 or 2 precooked 21DSD-approved breakfast sausages (see page 126), chopped

1 cup chopped romaine lettuce

2 or 3 pinches of Everything Bagel Spice Blend (page 248)

2 tablespoons Peanut Sauce (page 234), for serving

Heat the cooking fat in a small skillet over medium heat. Crack the eggs into the skillet and fry until the white is cooked but the yolk remains runny (or to your preferred level of doneness).

While the eggs are cooking, warm the sausage. You can do this in the same pan alongside the eggs, if desired, or in a separate skillet over medium heat.

Assemble the salad: Place the chopped lettuce on a plate and top with the egg, then garnish with the spice blend and add the sausage. Drizzle with peanut sauce to taste.

CHANGE IT UP

This recipe is almost infinitely flexible in the possible combinations of vegetable, meat, egg, and sauce. Below are some suggested swaps and additions.

- Arugula
- Sautéed kale
- Crispy Brussels Sprouts (page 194)
- Crispy Broccoli (page 200)
- Steamed green beans
- Roasted asparagus
- Zucchini noodles (page 174)
- Ranch Roasted Potatoes (page 206)
- Sautéed shredded sweet potato
- Simple Fried Rice (page 192)
- Poached eggs
- Scrambled eggs
- Crispy bacon
- Slow Cooker BBQ Pulled Pork (page 158)
- Avocado
- Green apple
- Salsa
- Pico de gallo
- Tahini Sauce (page 208)

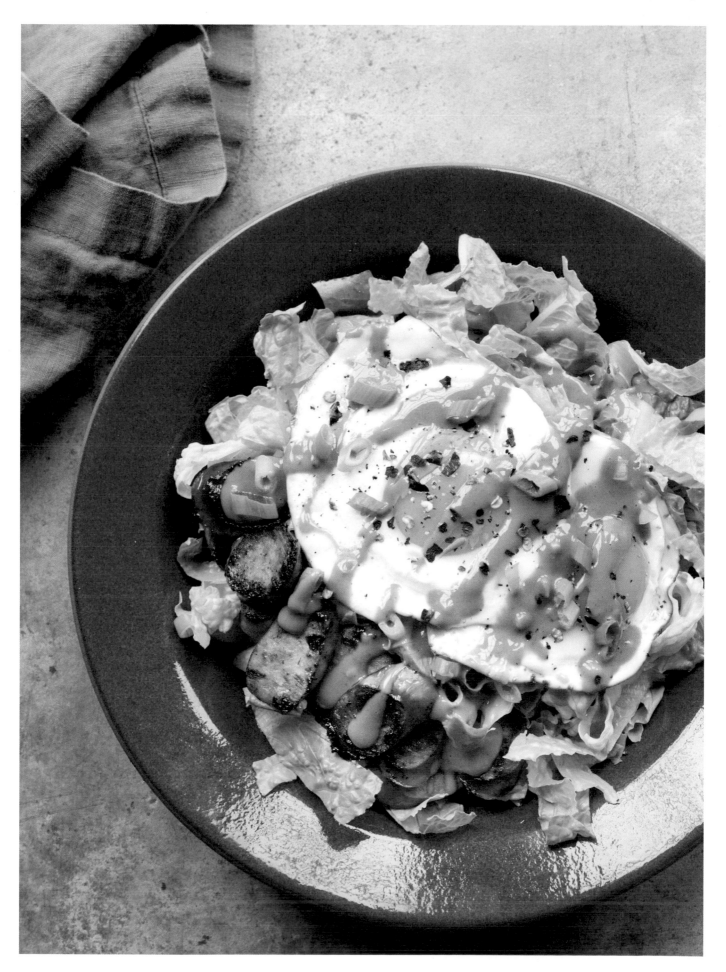

Apple Cinnamon Muffins

PREP TIME **20 MINUTES, PLUS 5 MINUTES TO CHILL THE APPLES** •
COOK TIME **35 MINUTES** • MAKES **12 LARGE MUFFINS (2 PER SERVING)**

NUTS
EGGS
NIGHTSHADES
FODMAPS

- 3 tablespoons coconut oil, divided
- 3 green apples, peeled and diced
- 9 eggs
- 1 1/2 teaspoons pure vanilla extract
- 3/4 cup + 3 tablespoons full-fat coconut milk, store-bought or homemade (page 243)
- 1 1/2 teaspoons apple cider vinegar
- 3/4 cup coconut flour, sifted
- 1 cup cashew flour, sifted
- 1 1/2 teaspoons baking soda
- 3 teaspoons ground cinnamon
- 1/4 teaspoon sea salt

Preheat the oven to 350°F. Line a 12-cavity muffin tin with parchment paper baking cups.

In a skillet over medium heat, melt 1 tablespoon of the coconut oil. Add the apples and sauté until soft, approximately 8 to 10 minutes. Place the cooked apples in the refrigerator to chill for at least 5 minutes.

In a large mixing bowl, vigorously whisk the eggs, vanilla, remaining 2 tablespoons of coconut oil, coconut milk, and vinegar for about 20 seconds, until combined. Add the coconut flour, cashew flour, baking soda, cinnamon, and salt to the egg mixture and whisk vigorously until smooth. Fold in the cooked and chilled apples.

Scoop the batter into the prepared muffin tin, filling each baking cup evenly. The muffins will be large and will puff up during baking, but they will deflate a bit once they cool.

Bake for 25 minutes, or until the muffins are puffed-up and golden brown. Store leftovers in an airtight container at room temperature for up to three days or in the refrigerator for up to a week.

21DSD FRUIT SERVING
Each muffin includes a quarter of a green apple (half a green apple per serving). Factor this into your total intake of allowed fruit for the day.

CHANGE IT UP
If you have Bob's Red Mill Paleo Flour on hand or want to use all almond flour, either of those will work for the flour in this recipe. Use 1 1/2 cups total.

If you have apple pie spice on hand, you can use 1 teaspoon apple pie spice and 2 teaspoons ground cinnamon instead of all cinnamon.

KITCHEN TIP
Parchment paper baking cups are critical to keep the muffins from sticking to the pan. They're easy to find at most grocery stores, or they can easily be ordered online on a site like Amazon. ●

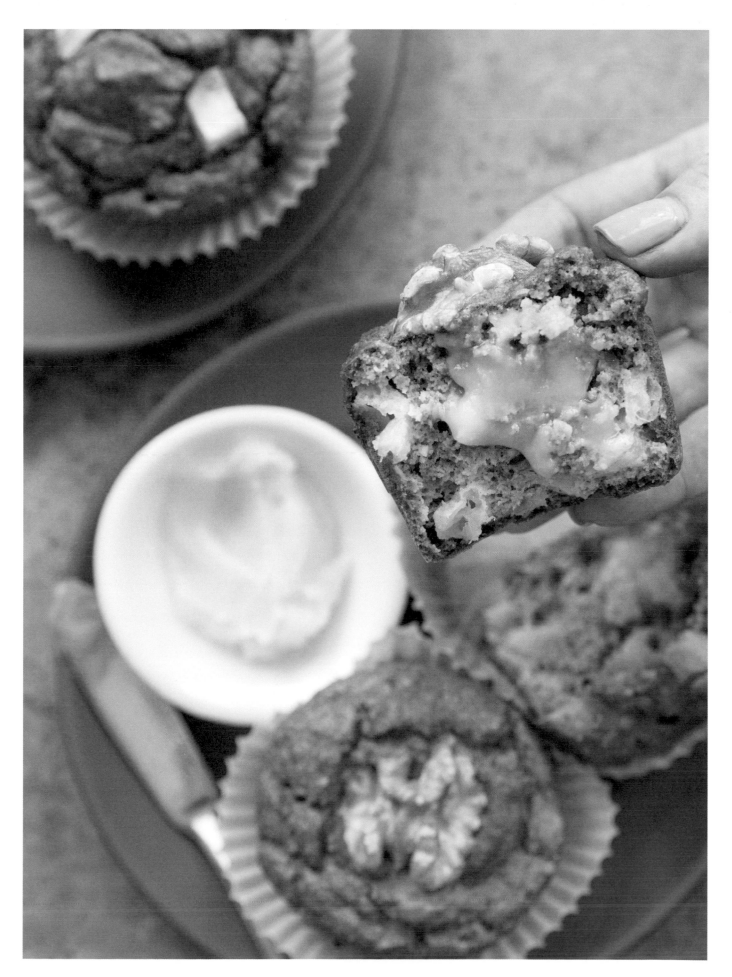

Mushroom, Pesto & Goat Cheese Frittata

PREP TIME **5 MINUTES, PLUS 20 MINUTES TO MAKE THE MUSHROOMS**
• COOK TIME **15 TO 20 MINUTES** • MAKES **2 SERVINGS**

NUTS

EGGS

NIGHTSHADES

FODMAPS

1 tablespoon cooking fat

1/2 cup Garlic Butter Sautéed Mushrooms (page 196)

4 eggs

2 tablespoons full-fat coconut milk, store-bought or homemade (page 243)

1/4 teaspoon sea salt

1/4 teaspoon ground black pepper or 1/2 teaspoon spice blend of choice (pages 248 to 249)

2 tablespoons Pesto Sauce (page 236)

2 ounces crumbled goat cheese (Levels 1 & 2 only)

Preheat the oven to 350°F.

Heat the cooking fat in an ovenproof 8-inch skillet over medium heat. Add the mushrooms and cook for 1 minute, to warm slightly.

While the mushrooms are cooking, whisk the eggs in a large bowl with the coconut milk, salt, and pepper. Add the egg mixture to the skillet and let set for 2 to 3 minutes. Top with the pesto and crumbled goat cheese, if using.

Transfer the skillet to the oven and bake for 10 to 15 minutes, until the eggs are no longer runny, the frittata puffs up a bit, and the edges are golden brown.

VARIATION: MUSHROOM, PESTO & GOAT CHEESE EGG MUFFINS

Line 4 cavities of a 12-cavity muffin tin with parchment paper baking cups. Divide the warmed mushrooms evenly among the muffin cavities, then pour in the egg mixture and top with the pesto and goat cheese, if using. Bake as instructed, but check after 10 minutes to make sure it doesn't overcook.

Parchment paper baking cups specifically are critical to ensure the eggs won't stick to the paper! They're easy to find at most grocery stores, or they can easily be ordered online on a site like Amazon.

KITCHEN TIP

If you don't have an 8-inch skillet, you can double the recipe and use a 10-inch skillet instead. Bake for 15 to 20 minutes. Store leftovers in the refrigerator for up to 5 days, or freeze individually wrapped portions for up to several weeks. Defrost in the refrigerator overnight before reheating, ideally in a toaster oven. ●

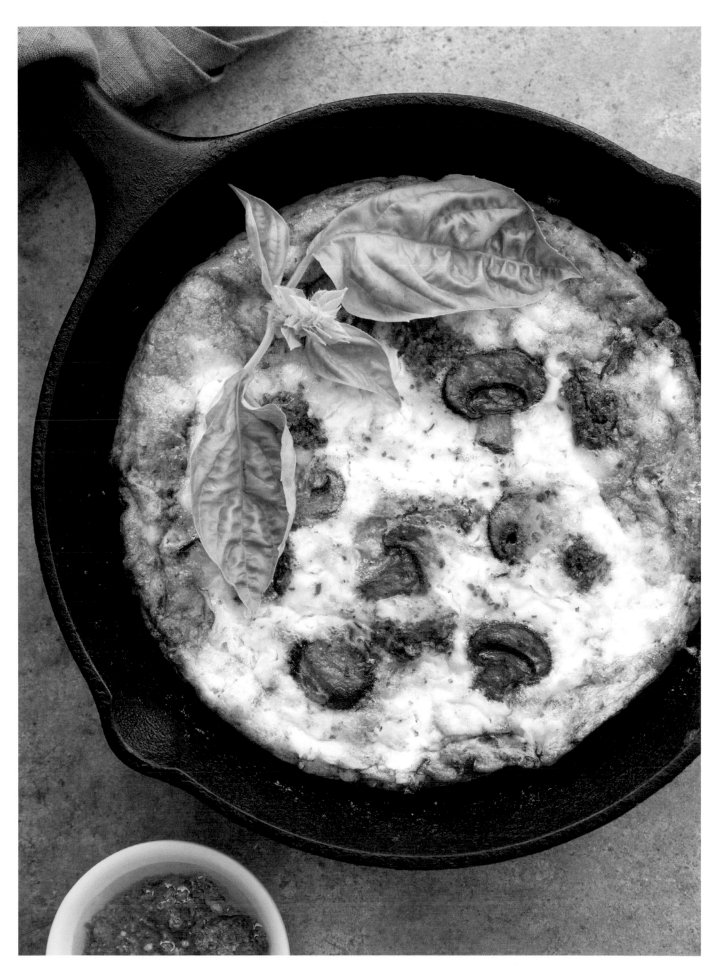

Broccoli, Ham & Cheese Frittata

PREP TIME **10 MINUTES, PLUS 30 MINUTES FOR THE CRISPY BROCCOLI**
• COOK TIME **15 TO 20 MINUTES** • MAKES **2 SERVINGS**

NUTS
EGGS
NIGHTSHADES
FODMAPS

1/2 pound cooked ham, cubed (see Note)

1/2 small red onion, chopped

4 eggs

2 tablespoons full-fat coconut milk, store-bought or homemade (page 243)

1/4 teaspoon sea salt

1/4 teaspoon ground black pepper or 1/2 teaspoon spice blend of choice (pages 248–249)

1 tablespoon cooking fat (optional)

1 cup Crispy Broccoli (page 200)

2 ounces cheddar cheese, grated (Levels 1 & 2 only)

Preheat the oven to 350°F.

Heat an ovenproof 8-inch skillet over medium heat. Add the ham and cook for 2 to 3 minutes to crisp slightly. Taste the ham—if it tastes fairly salty, use less salt later in the recipe. If the pan is looking a little dry, add the optional cooking fat.

Add the red onion, stir, and cook for 2 minutes.

While the onion is cooking, whisk the eggs in a large bowl with the coconut milk, sea salt, and black pepper. Add the egg mixture to the skillet and stir in the Crispy Broccoli and cheddar cheese, if using.

Bake for 10 to 15 minutes, until the eggs are no longer runny, the frittata puffs up a bit, and the edges are golden brown.

NOTE
Remember that 21DSD-friendly ham, bacon, and other cured meats may include sugar in the ingredients list as long as the amount of sugar listed in the Nutrition Facts is 0 grams. This is one of the few exceptions to the no-sweeteners rule. For more information, see page 126.

VARIATION: BROCCOLI, HAM & CHEESE EGG MUFFINS
Line 4 cavities of a 12-cavity muffin tin with parchment paper baking cups. Divide the cooked ham and onion, Crispy Broccoli, and cheddar cheese, if using, evenly among the prepared muffin cavities. Pour the egg mixture over the other ingredients. Bake according to the instructions, but check after 10 minutes to make sure it doesn't overcook.

Parchment paper baking cups specifically are critical to ensure the eggs won't stick to the paper! They're easy to find at most grocery stores, or they can easily be ordered online on a site like Amazon.

FODMAP-FREE?
Omit the onion.

KITCHEN TIP
If you don't have an 8-inch skillet, you can double the recipe and use a 10-inch skillet instead. Bake for 15 to 20 minutes. Store leftovers in the refrigerator for up to 5 days, or freeze individually wrapped portions for up to several weeks. Defrost in the refrigerator overnight before reheating, ideally in a toaster oven. ●

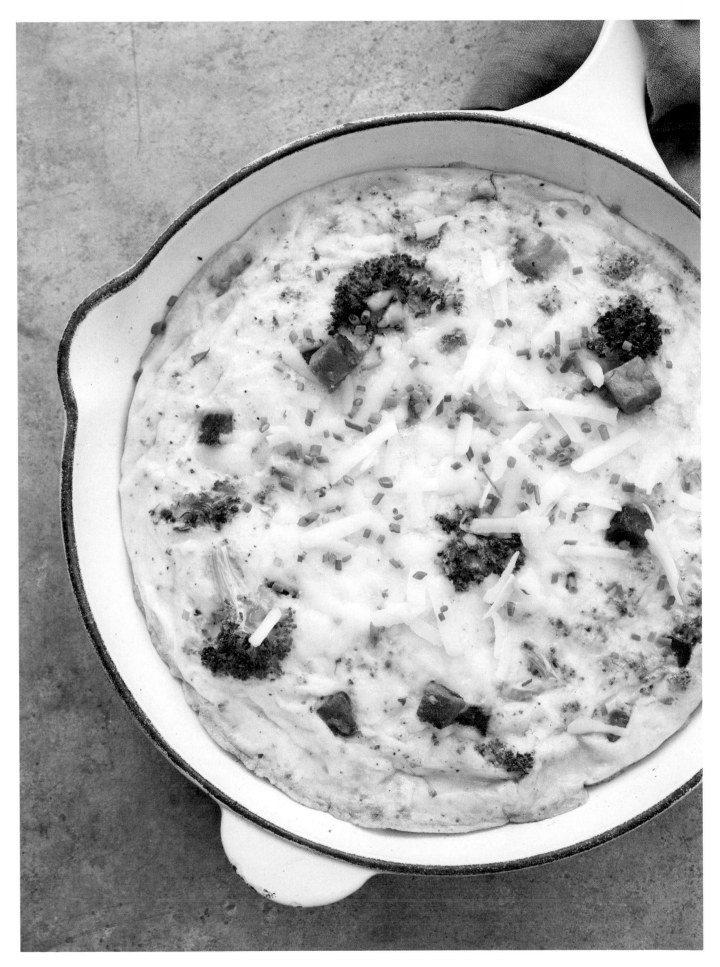

Sausage, Spinach & Peppers Frittata

PREP TIME **10 MINUTES** • COOK TIME **20 TO 25 MINUTES** • MAKES **2 SERVINGS**

NUTS
EGGS
NIGHTSHADES
FODMAPS

1/2 pound ground pork

2 tablespoons Italian Spice Blend (page 248)

1 red bell pepper, sliced

1 yellow bell pepper, sliced

1 small red onion, sliced

1 cup packed fresh spinach leaves

1/4 cup chopped fresh basil leaves

4 eggs

2 tablespoons full-fat coconut milk, store-bought or homemade (page 243)

1/4 teaspoon sea salt

1/4 teaspoon ground black pepper

Preheat the oven to 350°F.

Add the ground pork to an ovenproof 8-inch skillet over medium heat. As it begins to cook, add the Italian Spice Blend and cook for 5 minutes, or until no pink remains, breaking it up with a spatula as it cooks.

Add the peppers and onion to the skillet and cook until softened, about 3 to 4 minutes, then add the spinach and basil and cook for 1 minute to warm slightly.

While the sausage and vegetables are cooking, whisk the eggs in a large mixing bowl with the coconut milk, salt, and pepper.

Add the egg mixture to the skillet and bake for 10 to 15 minutes, until the eggs are no longer runny, the frittata puffs up a bit, and the edges are golden brown.

VARIATION: SAUSAGE, SPINACH & PEPPERS EGG MUFFINS
Line 4 cavities of a 12-cavity muffin tin with parchment paper baking cups. Divide the cooked sausage and vegetables evenly among the prepared muffin cavities. Pour the egg mixture over the other ingredients. Bake according to the instructions, but check after 10 minutes to make sure it doesn't overcook.

Parchment paper baking cups specifically are critical to ensure the eggs won't stick to the paper! They're easy to find at most grocery stores, or they can easily be ordered online on a site like Amazon.

KITCHEN TIP
If you don't have an 8-inch skillet, you can double the recipe and use a 10-inch skillet instead. Bake for 15 to 20 minutes. Store leftovers in the refrigerator for up to 5 days, or freeze individually wrapped portions for up to several weeks. Defrost in the refrigerator overnight before reheating, ideally in a toaster oven. ●

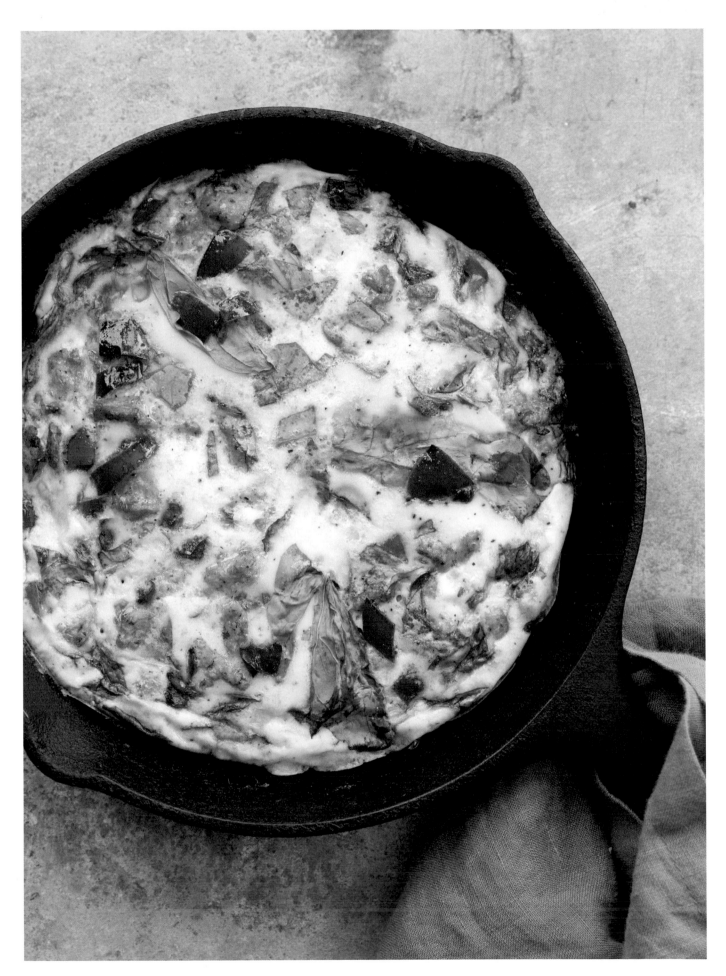

Bacon, Brussels, Asparagus & Goat Cheese Frittata

PREP TIME **10 MINUTES, PLUS 40 MINUTES FOR THE BRUSSELS SPROUTS** •
COOK TIME **16 TO 25 MINUTES** • MAKES **2 SERVINGS**

NUTS

EGGS

NIGHTSHADES

FODMAPS

1/2 pound bacon, chopped
(see page 126)

1 tablespoon cooking fat
(optional)

1/2 small red onion,
chopped

1/2 cup chopped fresh
asparagus (about 1-inch
pieces)

1 cup Crispy Brussels
Sprouts (page 194)

4 eggs

2 tablespoons full-fat
coconut milk, store-
bought or homemade
(page 243)

1/4 teaspoon sea salt

1/4 teaspoon ground black
pepper or 1/2 teaspoon
spice blend of choice
(pages 248–249)

2 ounces goat cheese,
crumbled (Levels 1 & 2
only)

Preheat the oven to 350°F.

Heat an ovenproof 8-inch skillet over medium
heat. Add the bacon and cook for 4 to 5 minutes to
render some of the fat. Taste the cooked bacon—if
it tastes fairly salty, use less salt later in the recipe.
If the pan is looking a little dry, add the optional
cooking fat.

Add the red onion to the skillet. Stir and cook for 2
minutes, then add the sliced asparagus and Crispy
Brussels Sprouts and allow to cook and warm
through for an additional 2 minutes.

While the vegetables are cooking, whisk the eggs
in a large bowl with the coconut milk, sea salt, and
pepper. Add the egg mixture to the skillet and top
with the goat cheese, if using.

Bake for 10 to 15 minutes, until the eggs are no
longer runny, the frittata puffs up a bit, and the
edges are golden brown.

VARIATION: BACON, BRUSSELS, ASPARAGUS & GOAT CHEESE EGG MUFFINS
Line 4 cavities of a 12-cavity muffin tin with parchment paper baking cups. Divide
the cooked vegetables evenly among the prepared muffin cavities. Pour the egg
mixture over the other ingredients and top with the goat cheese, if using. Bake
according to the instructions, but check after 10 minutes to make sure it doesn't
overcook.

Parchment paper baking cups specifically are critical to ensure the eggs won't
stick to the paper! They're easy to find at most grocery stores, or they can easily be
ordered online on a site like Amazon.

KITCHEN TIP
If you don't have an 8-inch skillet, you can double the recipe and use a 10-inch
skillet instead. Bake for 15 to 20 minutes. Store leftovers in the refrigerator for up to
5 days, or freeze individually wrapped portions for up to several weeks. Defrost in
the refrigerator overnight before reheating, ideally in a toaster oven.

FODMAP-FREE?
Omit the onion. ●

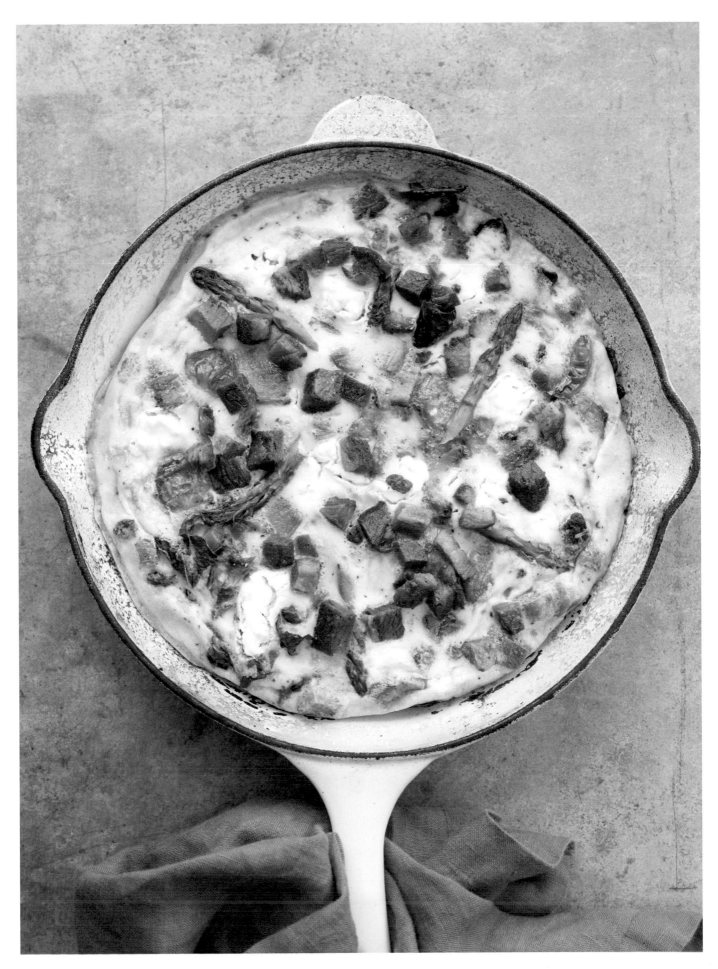

Banana Nut Smoothie

PREP TIME **5 MINUTES** • COOK TIME **—** • MAKES **2 SERVINGS**

NUTS

EGGS

NIGHTSHADES

FODMAPS

1 green-tipped banana, frozen

1 cup full-fat cashew or almond milk, store-bought or homemade (page 242)

1/2 cup water (optional)

1/4 cup almond butter

Seeds scraped from 1/4 vanilla bean pod or 1/2 teaspoon pure vanilla extract

1/4 teaspoon ground cinnamon

Small handful of ice (optional)

1 to 2 scoops protein powder (optional) (see Note)

Purée all the ingredients in a blender until smooth.

NOTE
Review the Yes/No Foods List (pages 19–21) for details on protein powder.

21DSD FRUIT SERVING
Each serving includes about half of a banana. Factor this into your total intake of allowed fruit for the day.

LOW-FODMAP?
You may find that green-tipped bananas work well for you (ripe bananas are higher in FODMAPs), or you can make this smoothie using 1/2 cup canned pumpkin instead of the banana. ●

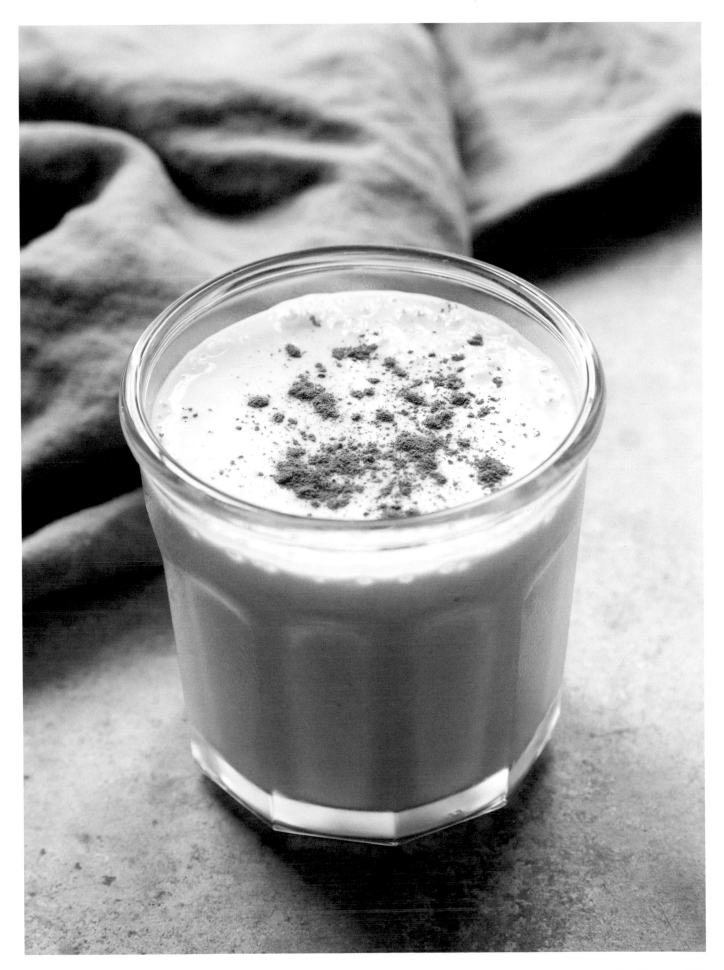

Apple Pie Smoothie

PREP TIME **10 MINUTES** • COOK TIME **—** • MAKES **2 SERVINGS**

NUTS

EGGS

NIGHTSHADES

FODMAPS

1 green apple, peeled, cored, and chopped

1 cup full-fat coconut milk, store-bought or homemade (page 243)

1/2 cup water

2 tablespoons almond butter

1 1/2 teaspoons ground cinnamon

1 teaspoon pure vanilla extract

Small handful of ice (optional)

1 to 2 scoops protein powder (optional) (see Note)

2 dashes nutmeg, for garnish

Purée all the ingredients in a blender until smooth. Garnish with nutmeg before serving.

NOTE
Review the Yes/No Foods List (pages 19–21) for details on protein powder.

21DSD FRUIT SERVING
Each serving includes about half of a green apple. Factor this into your total intake of allowed fruit for the day.

NUT-FREE?
Use coconut butter instead of almond butter. ●

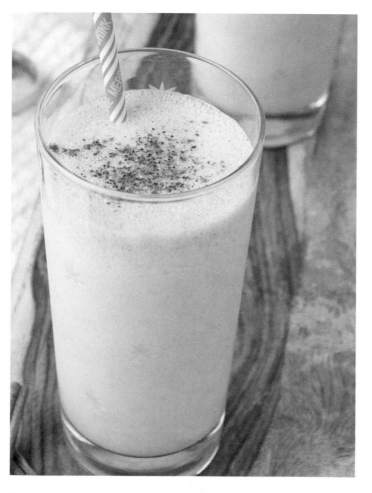

Pumpkin Spice Smoothie

PREP TIME **5 MINUTES** • COOK TIME **—** • MAKES **2 SERVINGS**

BREAK-FAST

- 1 green-tipped banana, frozen
- 1 cup full-fat coconut milk, store-bought or homemade (page 243)
- 1/2 cup water
- 1/4 cup canned pumpkin
- 1 teaspoon pure vanilla extract
- 1 teaspoon ground cinnamon, plus more for garnish (optional)
- 1 teaspoon pumpkin pie spice
- Small handful of ice (optional)
- 1 to 2 scoops protein powder (optional) (see Note)

Purée all the ingredients in a blender until smooth. Garnish with ground cinnamon before serving, if desired.

NUTS

EGGS

NIGHTSHADES

FODMAPS

NOTE
Review the Yes/No Foods List (pages 19–21) for details on protein powder.

21DSD FRUIT SERVING
Each serving includes about half of a banana. Factor this into your total intake of allowed fruit for the day. ●

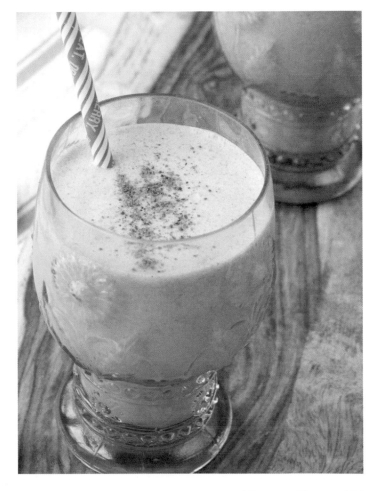

Banana Vanilla Bean N'Oatmeal

PREP TIME **15 MINUTES, PLUS 3 HOURS TO CHILL** •
COOK TIME **15 MINUTES** • MAKES **4 SERVINGS**

NUTS
EGGS
NIGHTSHADES
FODMAPS

2 eggs

1 vanilla bean pod

14.5 ounces coconut milk, store-bought or homemade (page 243) (about 1 3/4 cups)

1/2 cup water

1 medium green-tipped banana, sliced into coins

1 teaspoon ground cinnamon

Pinch of sea salt

1/4 cup chia seeds

Chopped nuts or banana slices, for garnish

Whisk the eggs in a small bowl and set the bowl next to your stove.

Slice the vanilla bean pod in half lengthwise, then, using the tip of a paring knife, scrape out the seeds. Put the scraped-out seeds, bean pod, coconut milk, and water in a saucepan and heat slowly over medium heat, stirring often. Once the mixture begins to simmer, stir more frequently; continue to simmer for 5 minutes. Remove the vanilla bean pod and discard.

Slowly pour a ladleful of the hot coconut milk mixture into the eggs as you whisk rapidly to incorporate. Then pour the coconut milk–egg mixture into the saucepan while continuing to whisk. Cook for 5 to 10 minutes, until a spoon remains coated when dipped into the mixture, stirring occasionally.

Pour the mixture into a blender, add the banana, and blend until smooth, approximately 1 to 2 minutes. Add the cinnamon, salt, and chia seeds and pulse a few times, until evenly mixed.

Divide the mixture into four serving bowls, jars, or glasses. Cover and refrigerate for at least 3 hours, preferably overnight.

Garnish with chopped nuts or banana slices. To serve warm, reheat in a saucepan over low heat until warmed through.

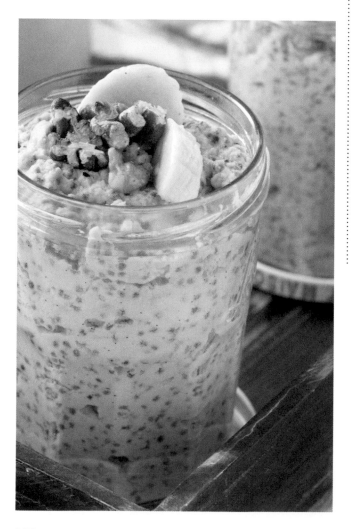

21DSD FRUIT SERVING
Each serving includes about a quarter of a banana. Factor this into your total intake of allowed fruit for the day.

EGG-FREE?
Omit the eggs. Blend all the ingredients in a blender, adding the chia seeds at the very end. Pour into containers and refrigerate for at least 4 hours. The consistency will be more like yogurt. ●

Grain-Free Banola

PREP TIME **10 MINUTES** • COOK TIME **30 TO 35 MINUTES** • MAKES **8 SERVINGS**

2 cups whole or halved nuts of choice (walnuts, pecans, macadamias, almonds)

1 cup slivered or sliced almonds

1/2 cup seeds of choice (pumpkin, sunflower, sesame)

1/2 cup almond meal, store-bought or homemade (page 242), or other nut meal

2 green-tipped bananas (to yield about 1 cup when puréed)

1 egg

2 teaspoons pure vanilla extract

2 teaspoons ground cinnamon

1/2 teaspoon nutmeg (optional)

1/4 teaspoon sea salt

NUTS

EGGS

NIGHTSHADES

FODMAPS

Preheat the oven to 350°F.

In a food processor, pulse the nuts until they're partially ground and partially still in small chunks. Pour the nuts into a large mixing bowl, then stir in the slivered almonds, seeds, and almond meal.

Place the bananas, egg, vanilla, cinnamon, nutmeg (if using), and sea salt into the food processor and process for 20 seconds or until all the ingredients are puréed. Pour the banana mixture into the nut mixture and stir until the nuts are well coated.

Pour the nut mixture onto a parchment paper–lined baking sheet.

Bake in the oven for about 30 to 35 minutes, checking every 10 minutes and turning the chunks of granola with a large spoon to break up the very large pieces. This allows it to dry out and lightly brown on all sides. Remove from the oven and let cool, uncovered, or turn off the oven and allow it to continue to dehydrate as the oven cools.

Store in an airtight container in the refrigerator for up to a week. Enjoy it plain as a snack, or with coconut or almond milk as a cereal.

21DSD FRUIT SERVING
Each serving includes about a quarter of a banana. Factor this into your total intake of allowed fruit for the day. ●

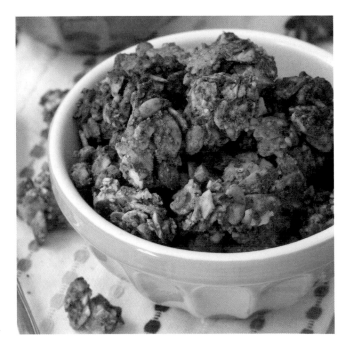

Bacon & Root Veggie Hash

PREP TIME **15 MINUTES** • COOK TIME **20 MINUTES** • MAKES **4 SERVINGS**

NUTS
EGGS
NIGHTSHADES
FODMAPS

4 slices bacon
1 shallot, minced
4 cups grated parsnips (approximately 8 medium)
1/4 cup grated carrots
1 tablespoon Italian Spice Blend (page 208)

Slice the bacon crosswise into 1/4-inch strips. In a large skillet over medium heat, cook the bacon until the fat is rendered and the meat is cooked, approximately 10 minutes. Remove the bacon from the pan and set on paper towels to drain, leaving the fat in the pan.

Add the shallot to the pan and cook for 2 minutes, or until it becomes translucent. Add the parsnips, carrots, and Italian Spice Blend to the pan and continue to cook until the vegetables are soft and cooked through, 5 to 8 minutes.

Add the bacon back to the pan and toss to combine and heat through.

Serve with eggs (any style) or your favorite breakfast sausage links.

FODMAP-FREE?
Omit the shallot. ●

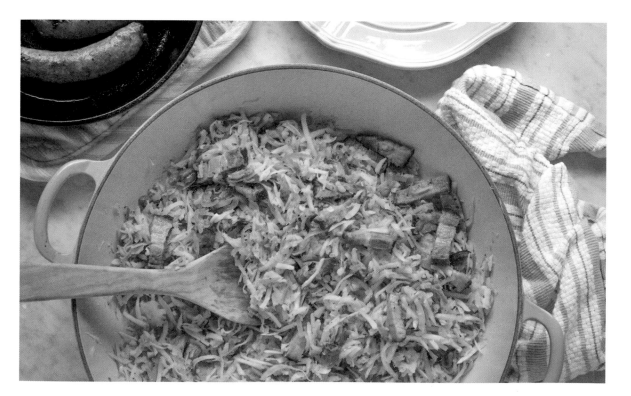

Pumpkin Pancakes
with Vanilla Bean Coconut Butter

PREP TIME **5 MINUTES** • COOK TIME **30 MINUTES** • MAKES **4 SERVINGS**

FOR THE PANCAKES

6 eggs

3/4 cup canned pumpkin

1 1/2 teaspoons pure vanilla extract

1 1/2 teaspoons pumpkin pie spice

1 1/2 teaspoons ground cinnamon

3 tablespoons coconut flour

1/4 teaspoon baking soda

Pinch of sea salt

3 tablespoons ghee or coconut oil, divided

FOR THE VANILLA BEAN COCONUT BUTTER

3 tablespoons coconut butter, softened

3/4 teaspoon pure vanilla extract

Seeds from 1/2 vanilla bean pod

NUTS

EGGS

NIGHTSHADES

FODMAPS

In a large mixing bowl, whisk the eggs, pumpkin, and vanilla. Sift the pumpkin pie spice, cinnamon, coconut flour, baking soda, and salt into the wet ingredients. Alternatively, pulse all the ingredients in a food processor until well mixed.

Grease a skillet with 1 teaspoon of the ghee and spoon the batter into the skillet to make pancakes of your desired size. Allow the pancakes to cook for about 3 minutes, and when a few bubbles appear, flip the pancakes and cook for another 3 minutes. Repeat with the remaining batter, greasing the pan each time.

Make the Vanilla Bean Coconut Butter: Combine the coconut butter, vanilla, and vanilla bean seeds in a small mixing bowl. Mix well to combine, then use to top the pancakes.

Serve with bacon or sausage.

CHANGE IT UP
Top with almond butter, sliced green-tipped bananas, or chopped walnuts or pecans.

KITCHEN TIP
If you are using freshly cooked or boxed pumpkin purée in this recipe, strain the excess water by placing it in cheesecloth over a bowl and refrigerate overnight before using it. ●

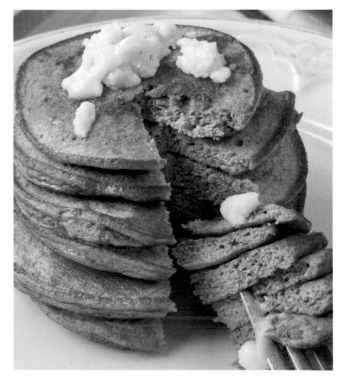

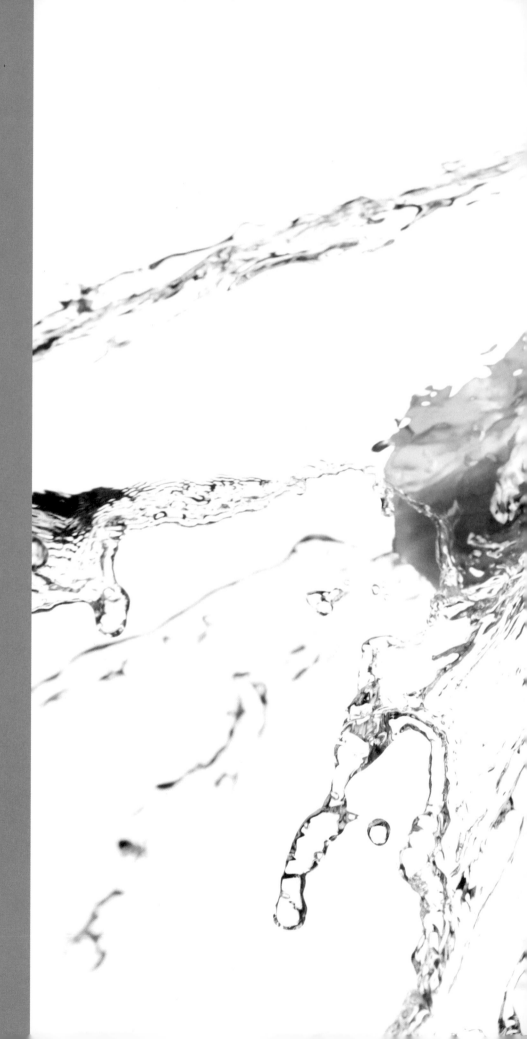

MAIN
DISHES

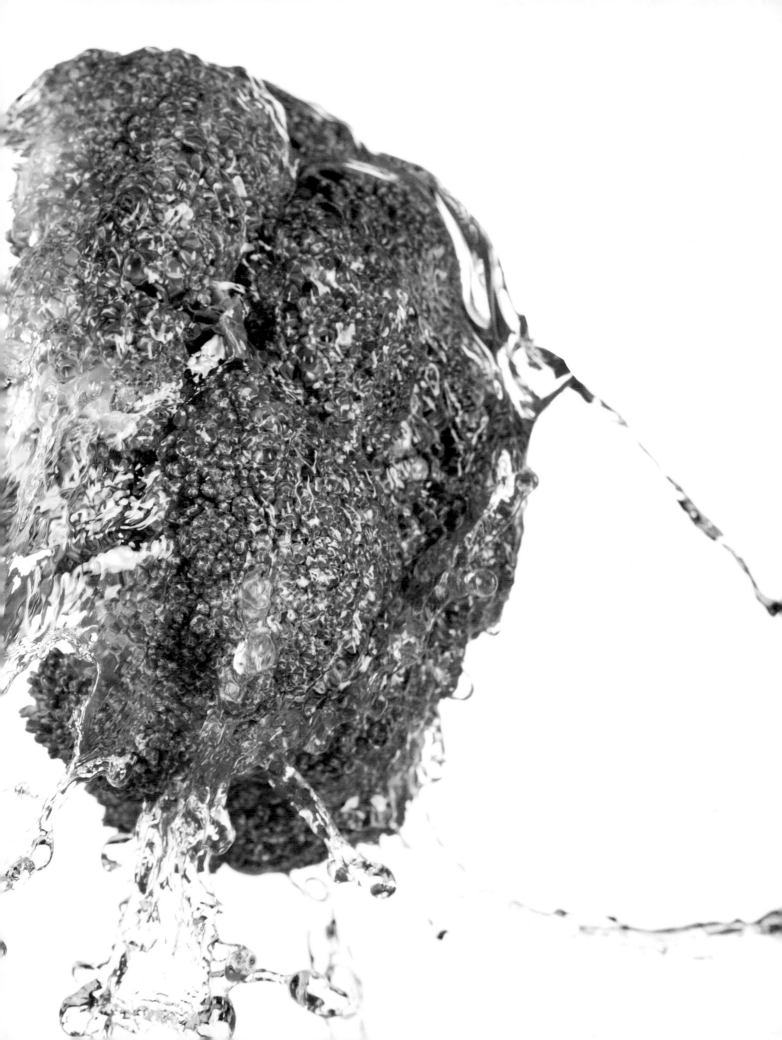

B3 Bowl

PREP TIME 5 MINUTES, PLUS 40 MINUTES TO MAKE THE BROCCOLI •
COOK TIME 10 TO 15 MINUTES • MAKES 2 SERVINGS

NUTS

EGGS

NIGHTSHADES

FODMAPS

1 tablespoon cooking fat

1 tablespoon Italian Spice Blend (page 248)

1/2 pound ground beef

1/2 pound ground pork

1 (24-ounce) jar sugar-free pasta sauce of choice

Sea salt and ground black pepper

1 batch Crispy Broccoli (page 200)

Fresh basil leaves, for topping (optional)

Grated cheese of choice, for topping (optional; Levels 1 & 2 only)

In a large skillet, melt the cooking fat over medium-high heat.

Season the beef and pork with the spice blend, then add the meat to the pan and cook until browned through, approximately 5 to 8 minutes.

Once the meat is done, add the pasta sauce and simmer over medium-low heat until the sauce is heated through, 5 to 10 minutes, stirring to combine.

Add salt and pepper to taste, then remove the pan from the heat.

Divide the Crispy Broccoli between two plates and ladle equal portions of the meat sauce over it. Garnish with fresh basil and grated cheese, if desired.

CHANGE IT UP
Try this served over Roasted Garlic Cauliflower Polenta (page 204) or Basic Cilantro Cauli-Rice (page 241). ●

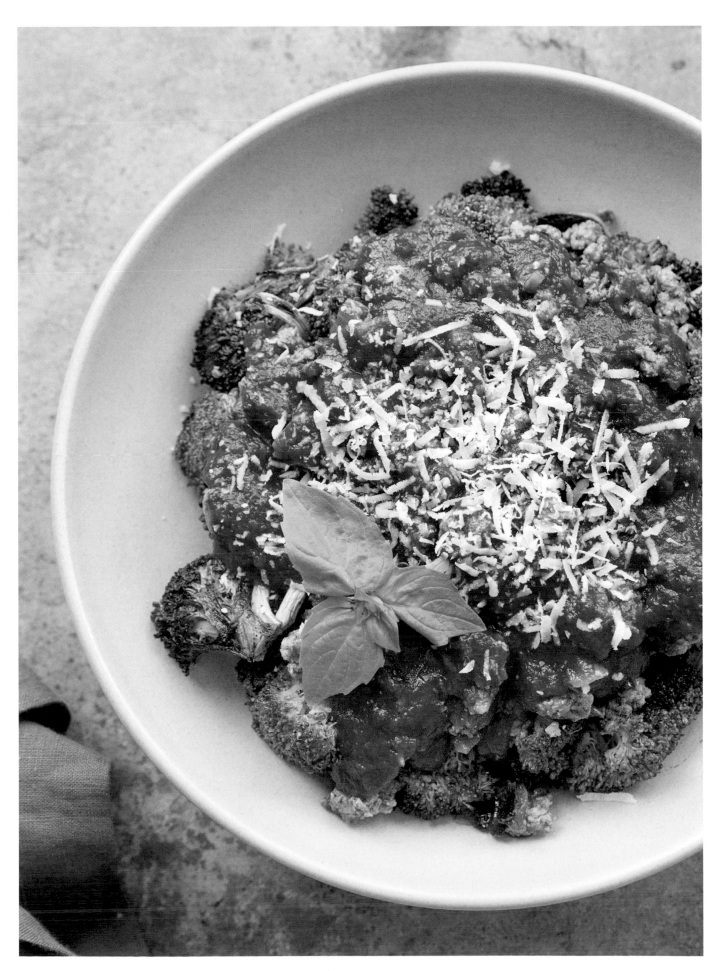

BBQ Burgers with Spicy Slaw

PREP TIME 15 MINUTES, PLUS 1 HOUR FOR CARAMELIZED ONIONS •
COOK TIME 15 MINUTES, PLUS 1 HOUR FOR CARAMELIZED ONIONS • MAKES 2 SERVINGS

NUTS

EGGS

NIGHTSHADES

FODMAPS

FOR THE SPICY SLAW

1 tablespoon extra-virgin olive oil

1 tablespoon red wine vinegar

1/4 teaspoon garlic powder

1/4 teaspoon onion powder

A few pinches of sea salt

A few pinches of ground black pepper

1 (16-ounce) bag coleslaw mix (or an equivalent amount of shredded cabbage and carrots)

1 jalapeño pepper, sliced, seeded if desired for less heat

1/2 pound ground beef

A few pinches of sea salt

A few pinches of ground black pepper

Grated or sliced cheddar cheese (see Note)

21DSD BBQ Sauce (page 233), for topping

Caramelized Onions (page 231), for topping

4 leaves butter lettuce, for serving

Make the slaw: In a large mixing bowl, combine the olive oil, vinegar, garlic powder, onion powder, salt, and pepper, and whisk until combined. Add the slaw mix and jalapeño and toss until the ingredients are evenly distributed.

Make the burgers: Preheat a grill or grill pan to medium-high heat.

In a mixing bowl, combine the ground beef with the salt and pepper and mix with your hands until well incorporated. Form the mixture into two patties.

Grill for 4 to 5 minutes per side to your desired level of doneness. Top the patties with the cheddar cheese and allow it to melt.

To serve, top the burgers with BBQ sauce, caramelized onions, and Spicy Slaw and wrap each in a lettuce leaf.

NOTE
If you're Level 3, replace the cheddar cheese with avocado slices.

KITCHEN TIP
For better flavor, chill the slaw in the refrigerator for at least an hour before serving. ●

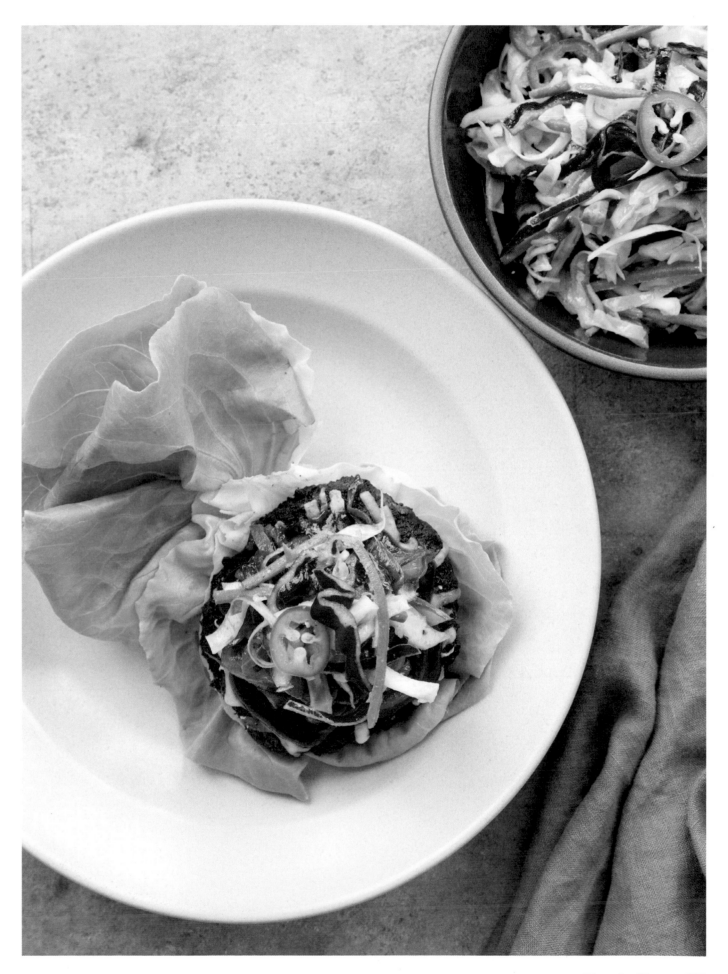

BBQ Chicken Salad

PREP TIME **15 MINUTES** • COOK TIME **45 TO 55 MINUTES** • MAKES **2 SERVINGS**

NUTS
EGGS
NIGHTSHADES
FODMAPS

2 pounds bone-in chicken thighs, with skin

3 tablespoons BBQ Spice Blend (page 248)

2 hearts of romaine lettuce, roughly chopped

1/4 red onion, sliced

1/4 cup chopped green onion

1/4 cup roughly chopped cilantro

2 tablespoons Smoky Toasted Almonds (page 212)

1/2 cup Ranch Dressing (page 240)

Preheat the oven to 375°F.

Season both sides of the chicken thighs with the spice blend. Place skin side up on a rimmed baking sheet and bake for 45 to 55 minutes, or until the internal temperature of the chicken reaches 165°F. Check the chicken after 15 minutes to make sure the spices aren't burning—if they look overly browned, brush some olive oil or fat on top of the thighs to moisten and cover with foil.

Remove the chicken from the oven and let it cool. Remove the skin and bone and chop into bite-sized pieces.

To serve, arrange the romaine lettuce hearts in a large serving bowl and top with the chicken pieces, red onion slices, green onion, cilantro, and almonds. Toss with or top with the dressing before serving.

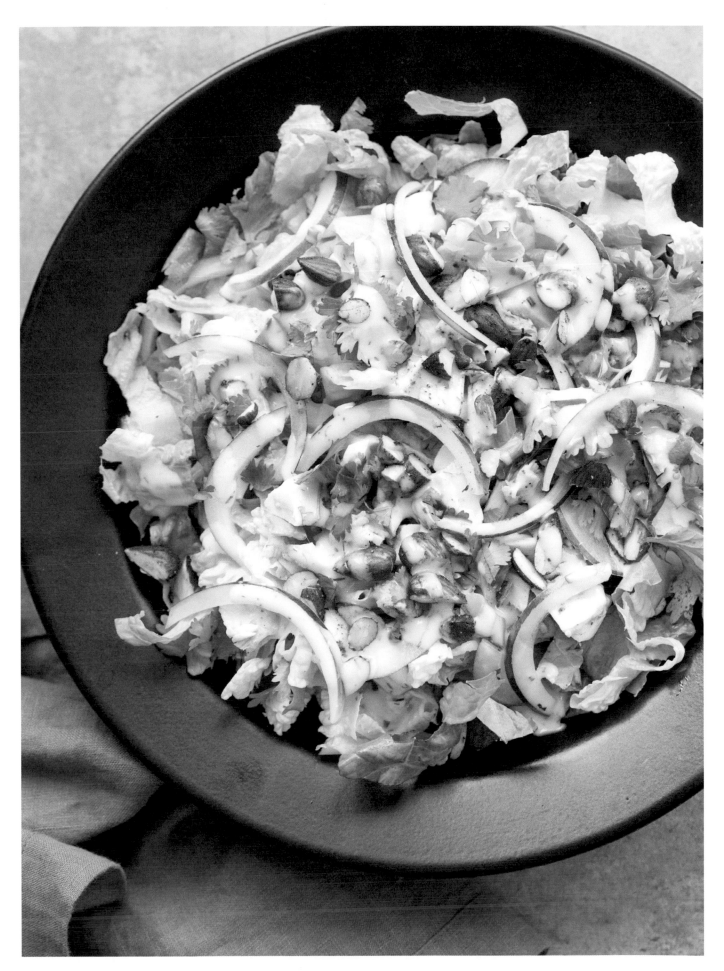

BBQ Pulled Pork Tacos with Spicy Slaw

PREP TIME **5 MINUTES** • COOK TIME **5 MINUTES**
• MAKES **6 LARGE OR 10 SMALL TACOS (2 SERVINGS)**

NUTS

EGGS

NIGHTSHADES

FODMAPS

This recipe comes together very quickly if you make the components ahead of time during a meal prep day. Allot 15 minutes prep time to make the pulled pork, spicy slaw, and marinated onions, and 6 to 8 hours in the slow cooker for the pork and to marinate the onions.

2 (4- to 6-ounce) servings Slow Cooker BBQ Pulled Pork (below)

6 large romaine lettuce leaves or 10 small butter lettuce leaves

1 cup Spicy Slaw (page 154)

1/2 cup Marinated Onions (page 176)

1/4 cup roughly chopped fresh cilantro

Ranch Dressing (page 240), for serving

In a medium skillet, warm the slow-cooker pork over medium-low heat.

Assemble the tacos: Using one lettuce leaf per taco, layer on the warmed pork, slaw, marinated onions, and cilantro. Serve with ranch dressing on the side.

CHEF TIP
Use two lettuce leaves per taco for less-messy tacos. ●

Slow Cooker BBQ Pulled Pork

PREP TIME **5 MINUTES** • COOK TIME **6 TO 8 HOURS** • MAKES **8 TO 10 SERVINGS**

NUTS

EGGS

NIGHTSHADES

FODMAPS

4 pounds pork shoulder roast

2 tablespoons BBQ Spice Blend (page 248)

1 cup chicken broth, store-bought or homemade (page 244)

10 cloves garlic, peeled

Season the pork shoulder liberally with the spice blend on all sides.

Place the meat, broth, and garlic cloves in a slow cooker and cook on low for 6 to 8 hours.

Remove the pork from the slow cooker and reserve any remaining liquid. Allow it to cool slightly, then shred it with two forks.

Taste the shredded meat and spoon more of the reserved liquid over it if needed for additional flavor.

Store in an airtight container in the refrigerator for up to 5 days.

NIGHTSHADE-FREE?
Use the Italian Spice Blend (page 248) on the pork instead of the BBQ Spice Blend.

KITCHEN TIP
To make this in an Instant Pot (electric pressure cooker), cut the pork into 2- to 3-inch pieces and cook on high pressure with 1 cup of water for 45 minutes. ●

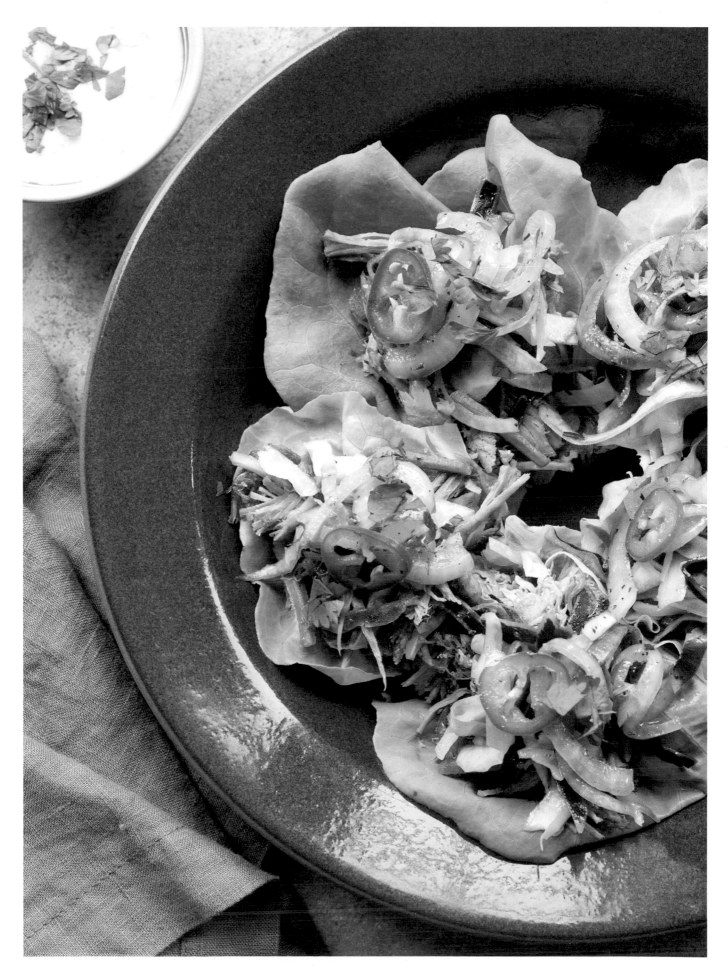

BBQ Pulled Pork Buddha Bowl

PREP TIME **5 MINUTES** • COOK TIME **5 MINUTES** • MAKES **2 SERVINGS**

NUTS

EGGS

NIGHTSHADES

FODMAPS

This recipe is a delicious and super-simple remix using items you'll have already made if you're following the daily meal plan. If you're not following the meal plan, allot 1 hour 30 minutes to make the cauli-rice, pulled pork, spicy slaw, marinated onions, and butternut squash, and 6 to 8 hours in the slow cooker for the pork and to marinate the onions.

The combination of flavors make eating this Buddha bowl, named for the balance of vibrant colors and bountiful healthy ingredients, a true delight.

2 cups Basic Cilantro Cauli-Rice (page 241)

1 cup Slow Cooker BBQ Pulled Pork (page 158)

1 cup Spicy Slaw (page 154)

1/2 cup Marinated Onions (page 176)

1/2 cup Roasted Butternut Squash (page 202), room temperature

21DSD BBQ Sauce (page 233)

1/4 cup chopped fresh cilantro, for garnish

Avocado slices, for garnish

In two small skillets, heat the cauliflower rice and pork over medium-low heat for about 5 minutes, just until warm.

Assemble the bowls: Ladle the warm cauliflower rice into two bowls. Top with the warmed pork, slaw, pickled onions, and butternut squash. Drizzle with BBQ sauce to taste and garnish with fresh cilantro and avocado slices.

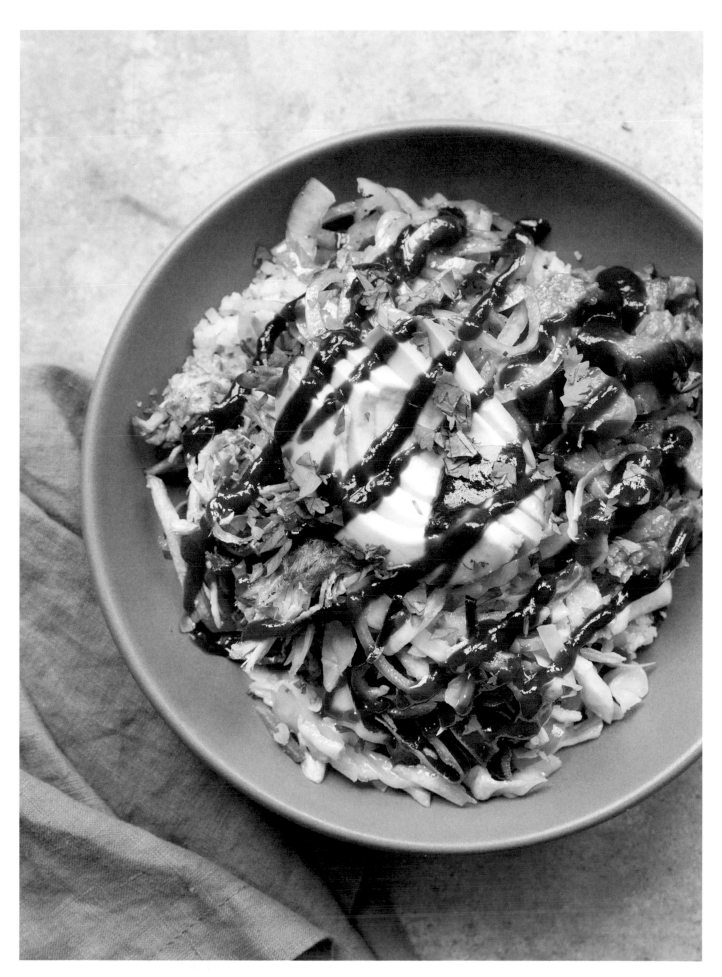

Buffalo Cauliflower & Chicken Wings

PREP TIME **10 MINUTES** • COOK TIME **50 MINUTES** • MAKES **2 SERVINGS**

NUTS

EGGS

NIGHTSHADES

FODMAPS

2 pounds chicken wings

2 medium to large heads of cauliflower, cut into florets

2 to 3 teaspoons Trifecta Spice Blend (page 249)

2 tablespoons chopped green onions, for garnish

FOR THE BUFFALO SAUCE

1/4 cup ghee

3 tablespoons sugar-free/sweetener-free hot sauce (see page 127)

FOR SERVING

Sliced carrots

Sliced celery

Ranch Dressing (page 240)

Preheat the oven to 375°F.

Season the wings and cauliflower generously with the Trifecta Spice Blend. Spread evenly on a baking sheet and bake for 50 minutes.

Make the Buffalo sauce: In a small bowl, combine the ghee and hot sauce and mix well.

Remove the wings and cauliflower from the oven. Toss with the Buffalo sauce and garnish with green onion. Serve with carrots, celery, and ranch dressing.

KITCHEN TIP
If you like your wings extra crispy, broil for two minutes before tossing with the Buffalo sauce. ●

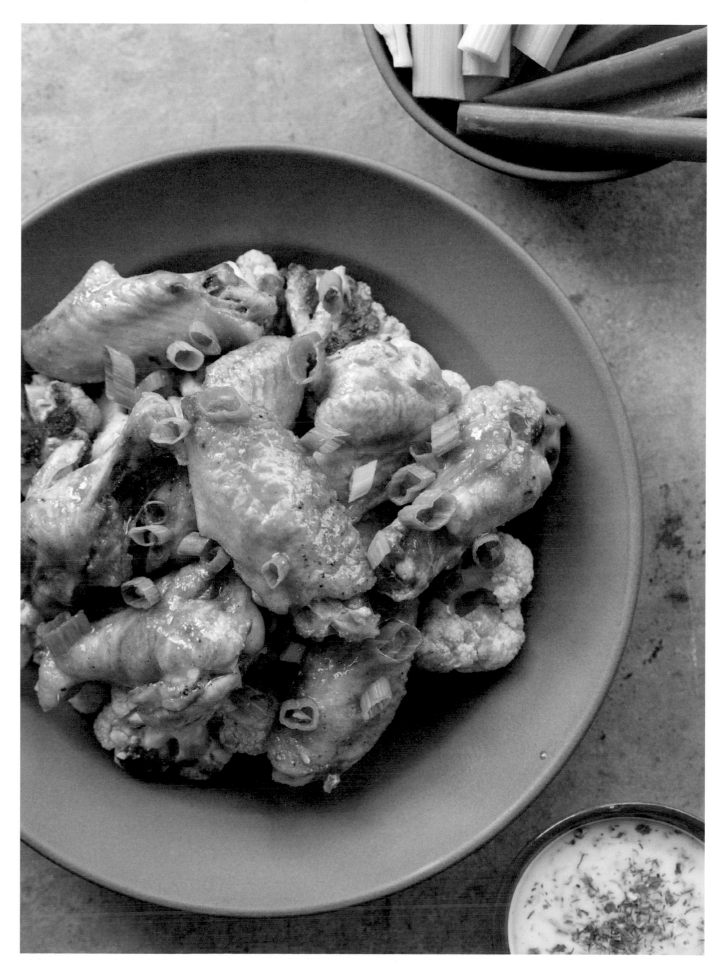

Chicken Fajita Salad

PREP TIME **15 MINUTES** • COOK TIME **14 TO 18 MINUTES** • MAKES **2 SERVINGS**

NUTS

EGGS

NIGHTSHADES

FODMAPS

3 teaspoons cooking fat, divided

1 red bell pepper, sliced into strips

1 yellow bell pepper, sliced into strips

1 small red onion, sliced into strips

2 chicken breasts (approximately 1 pound), cut into 1/4-inch strips

Sea salt and ground black pepper

1/4 cup + 2 tablespoons water, divided

1/2 teaspoon Taco & Fajita Spice Blend (page 249)

4 cups shredded romaine lettuce

1/2 avocado, sliced, for serving

2 tablespoons pico de gallo, for serving

1/4 cup chopped fresh cilantro, for serving

Juice of 1/2 lime, for serving

1/2 tablespoon extra-virgin olive oil, for serving

Heat 2 teaspoons of the cooking fat in a large skillet over medium-high heat. Add the veggies and stir, then let them sit a little to allow them to brown more easily. Cook for 5 to 7 minutes, until slightly browned and fork-tender. Remove from the skillet and set aside.

Season the chicken strips with salt and pepper. In the same skillet used to cook the veggies, melt the remaining teaspoon of fat over medium-high heat. Place the chicken strips in the hot skillet and sear each side. Depending on the size of your skillet, you may want to cook them in two batches so that they brown and cook through rather than steam as a result of an over-crowded pan.

Lower the heat to medium and continue to cook for 8 to 10 minutes, until the internal temperature of the chicken reaches 165°F.

Add 1/4 cup of the water to the pan and use a wooden spoon to scrape any brown bits from the bottom of the skillet.

Return the onions and peppers to the pan. Add the Taco & Fajita Spice Blend and the remaining 2 tablespoons of water. Stir to combine and heat through.

To serve, place the romaine lettuce in a large serving bowl and top with the chicken, onions and peppers, avocado, pico de gallo, and cilantro. Finish with the fresh lime juice, olive oil, and salt and pepper.

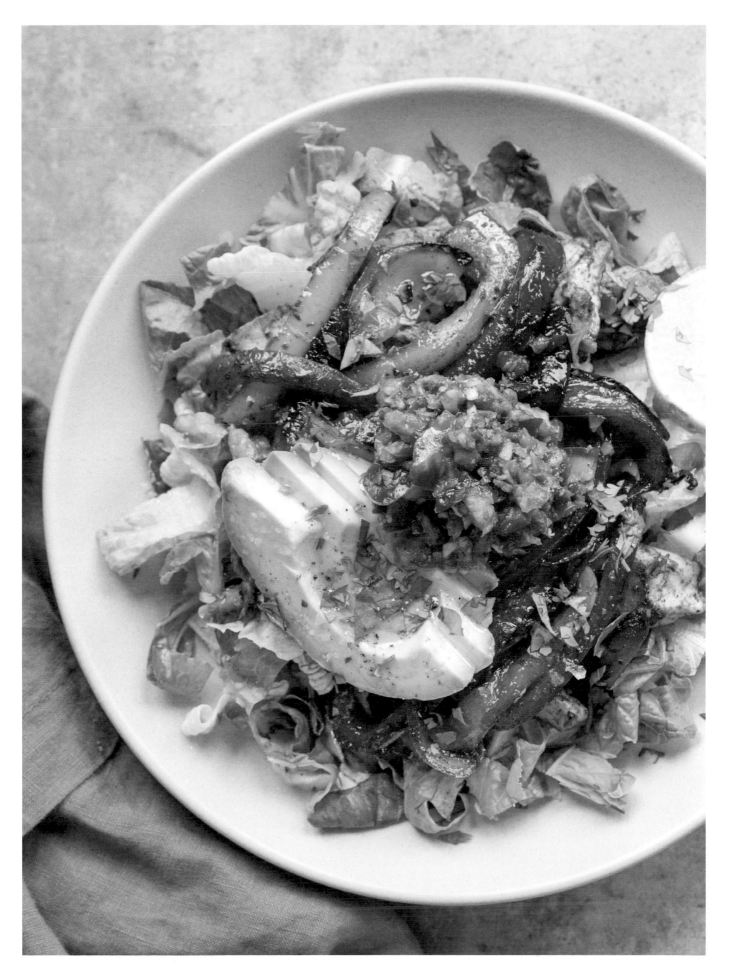

Ranch Chicken & Bacon Stuffed Potatoes

PREP TIME **15 MINUTES** • COOK TIME **1 HOUR** • MAKES **2 SERVINGS**

NUTS
EGGS
NIGHTSHADES
FODMAPS

2 large sweet potatoes

2 pounds chicken thighs, bone-in, with skin

3 tablespoons Ranch Spice Blend (page 249)

1 large head broccoli, cut into florets

1 tablespoon extra-virgin olive oil

2 slices bacon, chopped (see page 126)

1/2 cup Ranch Dressing (page 240), for serving

2 tablespoons chopped fresh chives, for garnish

CHANGE IT UP
Looking for a non-potato option? Serve with Roasted Garlic Cauliflower Polenta (page 204) or riced cauliflower instead! ●

Preheat the oven to 375°F.

Poke a few holes in the sweet potatoes with a fork, wrap in foil, and place in an oven-safe dish. Bake for 45 to 60 minutes, until fork-tender.

Season both sides of the chicken thighs with the spice blend and place skin side up on a rimmed baking sheet. Place in the oven with the sweet potatoes and bake for 35 to 45 minutes, until the internal temperature of the chicken reaches 165°F. Check after 15 minutes to make sure the spices aren't burning—if they look overly browned, brush some olive oil or other cooking fat on top of the thighs to moisten and cover with foil to finish baking.

As soon as the chicken goes into the oven, on a separate rimmed baking sheet, toss the broccoli florets with the olive oil and sprinkle with the bacon. Bake for 35 minutes alongside the chicken.

After the chicken is cooked, if desired, turn the oven to the broil setting and crisp the skin by broiling for 2 to 3 minutes.

Let the chicken cool slightly, then chop into bite-sized pieces. Discard the bones or freeze for up to several months for use in bone broth (page 244).

In a large mixing bowl, toss the chicken pieces with the broccoli and bacon.

Cut the sweet potatoes in half lengthwise and stuff with the chicken-broccoli mixture. Dress with ranch dressing and garnish with chives before serving.

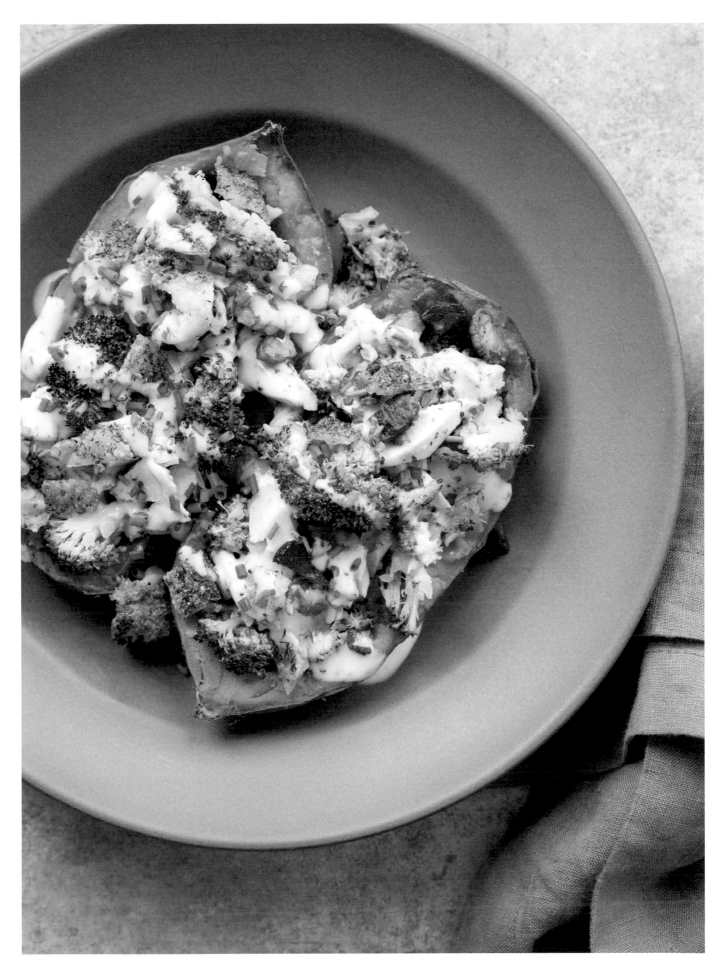

Cheesesteak Stuffed Potatoes

PREP TIME **15 MINUTES** • COOK TIME **40 TO 60 MINUTES** • MAKES **2 SERVINGS**

NUTS

EGGS

NIGHTSHADES

FODMAPS

2 large potatoes, white or sweet

1 pound skirt steak, flank steak, or chicken breast

Trifecta Spice Blend (page 249)

2 teaspoons cooking fat

1 green bell pepper, sliced into strips

1 small yellow onion, sliced into strips

Sea salt and ground black pepper

Cashew "Cheese" Sauce (page 235), for serving

Preheat the oven to 350°F. Use a fork to poke several holes in each potato, then wrap each potato in foil. Place on a sheet pan and bake for 40 to 50 minutes, until fork-tender.

While the potatoes bake, make the steak and filling: Preheat a grill to medium-high heat. Season the steak liberally with the spice blend.

Grill for about 5 minutes per side, turning the steak 90 degrees halfway through cooking to achieve crosshatch grill marks. Set the cooked steak aside to rest.

In a large skillet over medium-high heat, melt the cooking fat. Add the bell pepper and onion and season with salt and pepper. Sauté for 8 to 10 minutes, until soft and slightly browned on the edges. Remove from the heat and set aside.

Cut the steak into 1/4-inch slices, cutting on a slight angle against the grain.

Cut the baked potatoes in half lengthwise. Top each potato half with slices of steak, peppers, and onions. Drizzle with "cheese" sauce and serve.

CHANGE IT UP
If you're looking for a non-potato option, serve with Roasted Garlic Cauliflower Polenta (page 204) or riced cauliflower instead!
Doing Level 1 or 2 of the 21DSD? Feel free to melt full-fat cheese on top of these instead of the "cheese" sauce. I'd suggest provolone for this recipe. ●

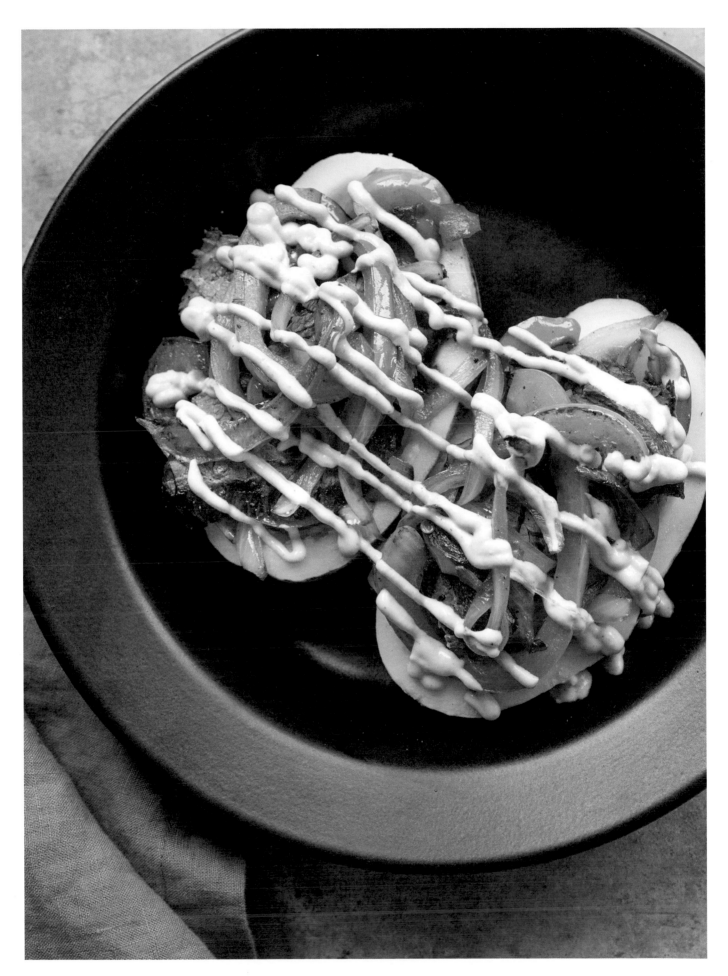

Diane's Simple Roast Chicken

PREP TIME **10 MINUTES** • COOK TIME **1 HOUR 10 MINUTES** • MAKES **4 TO 6 SERVINGS**

NUTS

EGGS

NIGHTSHADES

FODMAPS

2 medium yellow onions, roughly chopped

4 tablespoons cooking fat, divided

2 to 3 pinches of sea salt

2 to 3 pinches of ground black pepper

2 to 3 pinches of garlic powder

1 teaspoon dried ground oregano or 2 to 3 pinches of Greek Spice Blend (page 248)

1 whole chicken, about 3 1/2 to 4 pounds

FODMAP-FREE?
In place of the onions, use 4 large carrots, peeled and sliced into 1/2-inch coins.

KITCHEN TIP
Save the bones from your chicken to make bone broth (page 244). ●

Preheat the oven to 375°F.

Place the onions in a large roasting pan. Add 2 tablespoons of the cooking fat, the salt, pepper, garlic powder, and oregano, and toss to combine.

Place the chicken on the onions, breast side up. Tie the chicken legs together with kitchen string. If you like, cut a small slit next to each leg and tuck the wing tip into it to keep the tips from overly browning or burning.

Brush the chicken with the remaining 2 tablespoons of cooking fat. Season generously with additional salt, pepper, garlic powder, and dried oregano.

Roast for 60 minutes, or until the internal temperature of the chicken reaches 165°F. (Test the temperature by inserting the thermometer into a meaty part of the leg, avoiding the bone.)

Remove the chicken from the oven and transfer it to a cutting board (keep the onions in the pan). Let the chicken rest for at least 10 minutes.

While the chicken rests, return the onions in the roasting pan to the oven for 10 minutes, or until caramelized, stirring once to ensure they're evenly coated with any drippings from the chicken.

Serve the roasted onions with the chicken.

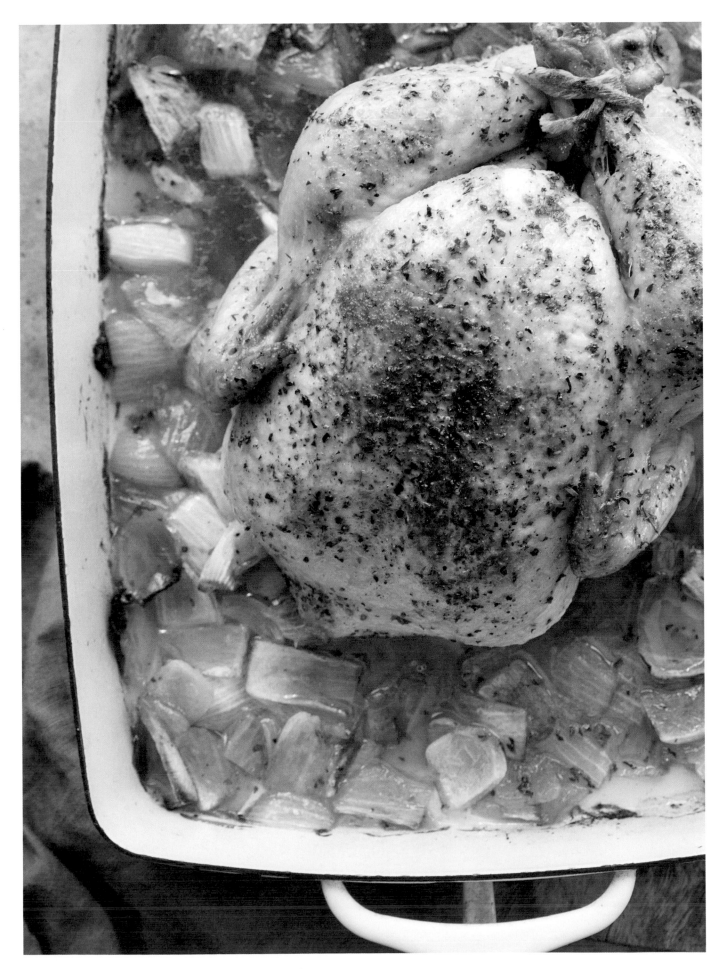

Smoky Chicken Salad Lettuce Boats

PREP TIME **10 MINUTES, PLUS TIME TO COOK THE CHICKEN** •
COOK TIME — • MAKES **2 SERVINGS**

NUTS

EGGS

NIGHTSHADES

FODMAPS

2 tablespoons mayonnaise, store-bought or homemade (page 246)

1/2 teaspoon Smoky Spice Blend (page 248)

1/4 cup finely chopped celery

1/4 cup finely chopped red onion

8 ounces chicken breast, cooked and shredded or finely chopped

Sea salt and ground black pepper

4 leaves romaine lettuce

Sliced tomato, for serving

In a medium mixing bowl, combine the mayonnaise, spice blend, celery, and red onions.

Add the shredded chicken and mix to combine. Taste to check the seasoning and add salt and pepper if needed.

Serve in romaine lettuce leaves and garnish with tomato slices and an extra sprinkling of the spice blend and black pepper.

EGG-FREE?
Mash half of a ripe avocado to use in place of the mayonnaise. ●

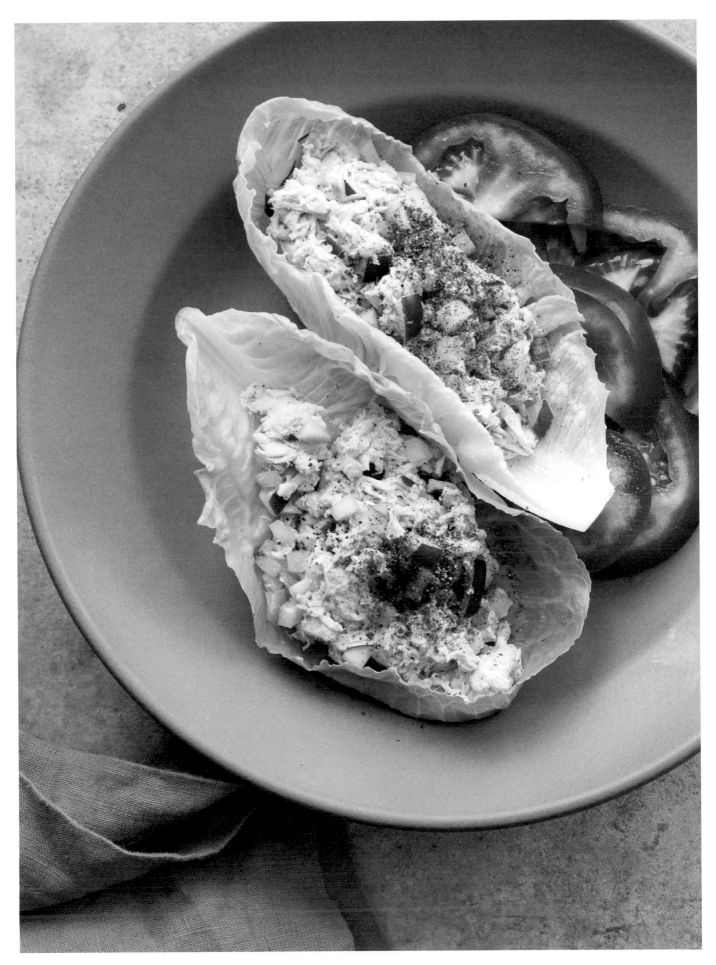

Creamy Mustard Chicken
with Zoodles

PREP TIME **15 MINUTES** • COOK TIME **25 MINUTES** • MAKES **2 SERVINGS**

NUTS
EGGS
NIGHTSHADES
FODMAPS

2 large or 4 small zucchini

1 pound boneless, skinless chicken thighs, or 2 pounds bone-in chicken thighs, cut into bite-sized pieces

2 tablespoons cooking fat, divided

Trifecta Spice Blend (page 249)

1 to 2 cloves garlic, minced or grated

1 pound mushrooms, sliced

Pinch of sea salt

Pinch of black pepper

1/2 cup chicken broth, store-bought or homemade (page 244)

1/2 cup full-fat coconut milk, store-bought or homemade (page 243)

1 teaspoon onion powder

1 tablespoon Dijon mustard

Grated Parmesan, Romano, or other hard cheese of choice, for garnish (optional; Levels 1 & 2 only)

Fresh chives, chopped, for garnish (optional)

Make the zucchini noodles: Fill a large pot with 1 inch of water, cover, and bring to a boil over high heat. Place a steamer basket in the pot.

While the water comes to a boil, shred the zucchini or yellow squash into noodles using a handheld julienne peeler, a spiralizer tool, or even a regular vegetable peeler (if using a regular peeler, the noodles will be wide and flat instead of spaghetti-shaped). You should get 2 cups of noodles.

When the water is boiling, steam the noodles in the basket for 3 minutes, then place them in a colander to drain off the excess liquid as they cool slightly. Set aside.

Make the chicken: In a large skillet over medium heat, melt 1 tablespoon of the cooking fat. Place the chicken in the pan and cook for about 5 minutes. Season liberally with the spice blend halfway through cooking. Remove the chicken from the pan and set aside.

In the same skillet, add the remaining tablespoon of cooking fat and increase the heat to medium-high. Add the garlic and stir for 30 seconds. Add the mushrooms, salt, and pepper and stir to coat. Let sit for 2 to 3 minutes, stir again, and then cook for 7 to 8 minutes, until fork-tender.

Lower the heat to medium, add the chicken, and toss to coat. Season with additional salt and pepper to taste, then add the broth, coconut milk, onion powder, and mustard. Stir to combine, then lower the heat to medium-low and simmer for 2 to 3 minutes, until the sauce has mostly been absorbed into the mushrooms and chicken.

Serve over the zucchini noodles and garnish with grated cheese and chives, if desired.

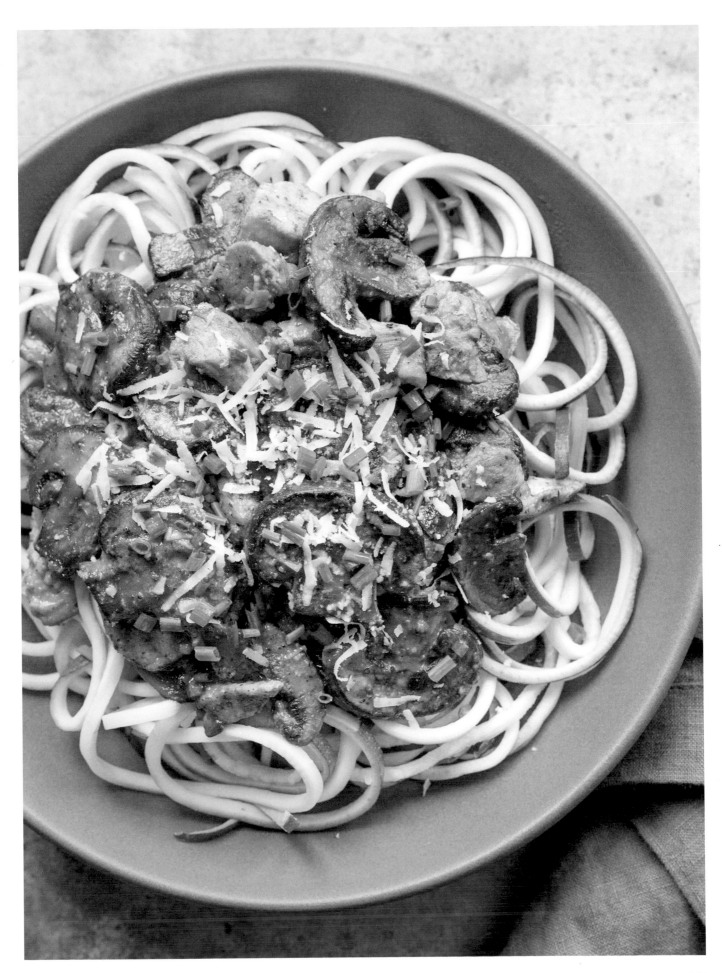

Tangy Chicken Salad

PREP TIME **20 MINUTES, PLUS OVERNIGHT TO MARINATE THE ONIONS** •
COOK TIME **—** • MAKES **2 SERVINGS**

NUTS

EGGS

NIGHTSHADES

FODMAPS

**FOR THE MARINATED ONIONS
(MAKES ABOUT 2 CUPS)**

1/4 cup extra-virgin olive oil

1/4 cup red wine vinegar

1 1/2 teaspoons sea salt

1 teaspoon dried oregano

1/2 teaspoon garlic powder

1/4 teaspoon ground black
pepper

2 medium red onions, cut in
1/4-inch-thick half moons

2 cups roughly chopped
kale

2 cups roughly chopped
romaine lettuce

1/2 cup sliced fennel

1/2 pound roast chicken,
shredded

1 ruby red grapefruit,
segmented

1/2 cup fresh pea shoots
or other micro greens or
sprouts (optional)

4 ounces full-fat mizithra,
feta cheese, or goat
cheese (Levels 1 & 2 only)

1/2 cup Ranch Dressing
(page 240)

Make the onions: In a medium-sized mixing bowl,
mix together the oil, vinegar, and spices. Add
the onions, cover, and marinate overnight in the
refrigerator.

Make the salad: In a serving bowl, toss the kale,
romaine lettuce, fennel, and shredded chicken
together with the dressing. Top with the marinated
onions, grapefruit segments, pea shoots, if using,
and cheese.

IF YOU'RE FOLLOWING THE MEAL PLAN
Since you're eating just one serving of salad,
only use half the amount of dressing; reserve
the other half and toss it with the second
serving of salad just before you eat it.

KITCHEN TIP
To segment your citrus fruit: Using a sharp
paring knife, slice along the outer curve
of the fruit, carefully removing all of the
skin and white pith. Next, carefully slice
diagonally from the outside toward the
center of the fruit, running the knife next to
each thin piece of divider skin to remove the
fleshy portions in between. The segments
will slide out cleanly.

AFTER THE 21DSD
Use an orange instead of a grapefruit
once you have completed the 21DSD for a
naturally sweet option!

NIGHTSHADE-FREE?
Omit the red pepper flakes. ●

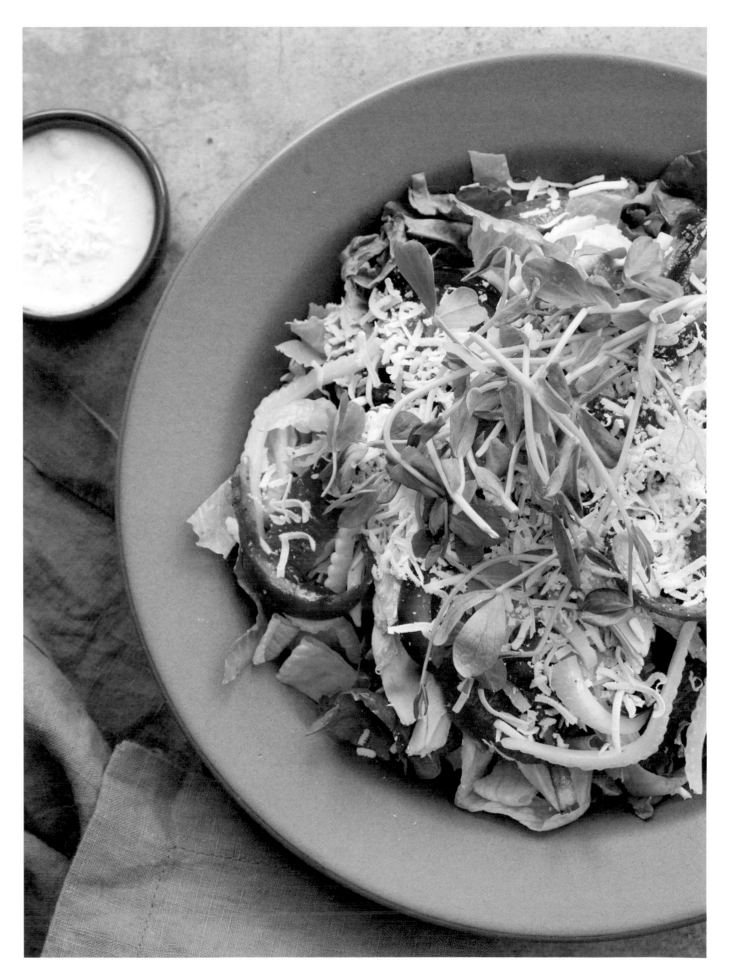

Deli Tuna Sliders

PREP TIME **15 MINUTES** • COOK TIME — • MAKES **2 SERVINGS**

NUTS

EGGS

NIGHTSHADES

FODMAPS

1 medium carrot, peeled

1/2 small red onion

2 (6-ounce) cans tuna (reserve the liquid)

4 to 6 tablespoons mayonnaise, store-bought or homemade (page 246)

1 teaspoon Trifecta Spice Blend (page 249)

1/4 cup finely chopped celery

6 leaves butter lettuce

Red onion slices, for serving

Tomato slices, for serving

Fit your food processor with the shredding blade and shred the carrot and red onion. Alternatively, shred them by hand with a box grater.

Add the tuna and 1/2 tablespoon of the liquid from the can, the mayonnaise, and the spices. If you prefer creamier tuna salad, use more mayonnaise.

Pulse 6 to 10 times, until well combined. Add in the celery and stir to combine.

If you do not have a food processor, combine all the ingredients but the lettuce leaves in a large mixing bowl and stir to mix well.

Taste and add additional seasoning if desired.

Place the tuna on lettuce leaves (you can layer two leaves if you like) and serve with slices of red onion and tomato.

EGG-FREE?
Mash half of a ripe avocado to use in place of the mayonnaise.

NIGHTSHADE-FREE?
Omit the tomato slices. ●

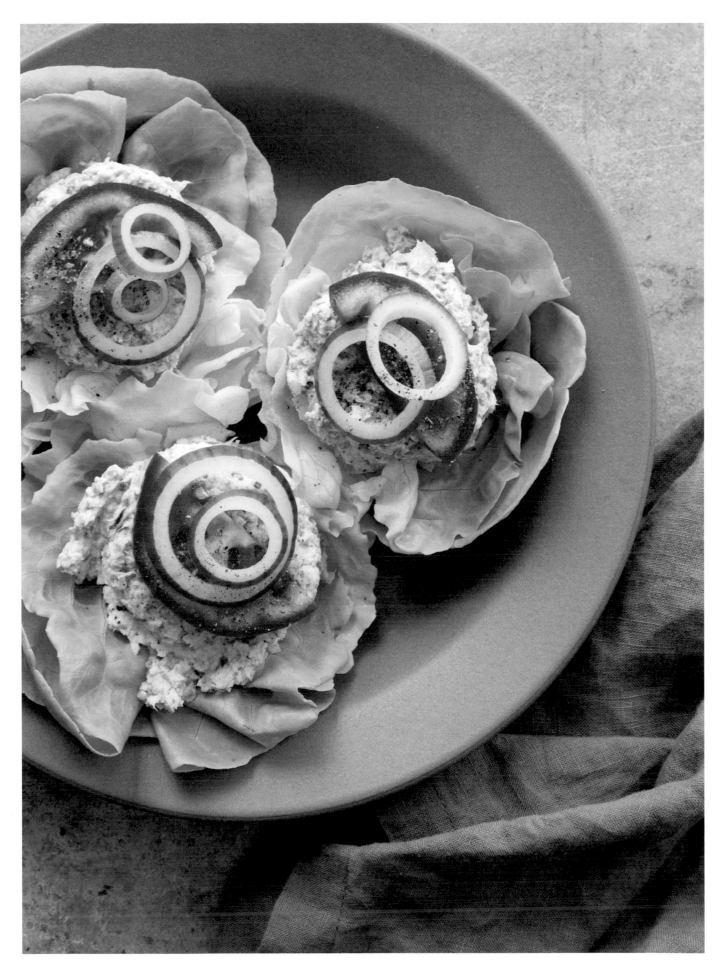

Mediterranean Meatball Bowl

PREP TIME **20 MINUTES, PLUS 55 MINUTES FOR THE EGGPLANT AND TAHINI SAUCE** •
COOK TIME **25 TO 30 MINUTES** • MAKES **2 SERVINGS**

NUTS

EGGS

NIGHTSHADES

FODMAPS

FOR THE MEATBALLS

1/2 cup chopped fresh cilantro, basil, or mint (or any combination) (reserve 1 tablespoon for garnish)

2 cloves garlic, grated or minced

1/2 teaspoon sea salt

1/2 teaspoon ground black pepper

1 pound ground lamb or beef

FOR THE TABBOULEH

3 tablespoons extra-virgin olive oil, divided

1 (12-ounce) package riced cauliflower (see page 127)

1 teaspoon garlic powder

1 teaspoon dried oregano

Pinch of sea salt

Pinch of ground black pepper

1 tomato, chopped

1 medium cucumber, chopped

1/4 small red onion, sliced

1/2 lemon

1/4 cup Kalamata olives, whole or sliced

1 serving Roasted Eggplant Steaks (page 208), chopped

Tahini Sauce (page 208), for garnish

Lemon wedges, for garnish

Preheat the oven to 375°F. Line a rimmed baking sheet with foil, then place a wire baking rack on top of it.

Make the meatballs: In a large mixing bowl, combine the herbs, garlic, salt, and pepper. Add the meat and use your hands to thoroughly mix it with the seasonings. Form the seasoned meat into sixteen meatballs, about 1 ounce each (1 1/2 inches in diameter).

Place the meatballs on the prepared baking sheet and bake for 25 to 30 minutes, until cooked through.

While the meatballs are baking, make the salad: In a large skillet over medium heat, warm 1 tablespoon of the olive oil. Place the cauliflower rice in the skillet and add the garlic powder, oregano, salt, and pepper. Sauté for about 5 minutes, until the cauliflower begins to become translucent, stirring gently to ensure that it cooks through. Transfer the cauliflower rice to a serving bowl and let cool to room temperature.

Toss the cooled cauliflower rice with the tomato, cucumber, red onion, the remaining 2 tablespoons of olive oil, and a squeeze of lemon.

Top with the olives, eggplant, meatballs, and a drizzle of tahini sauce. Garnish with the reserved tablespoon of herbs and lemon wedges before serving.

CHANGE IT UP
Level 1 or 2? Feel free to add feta cheese or mizithra cheese.

NIGHTSHADE-FREE?
Omit the tomato and use twice the cucumbers for the salad, or replace the tomatoes with beets. ●

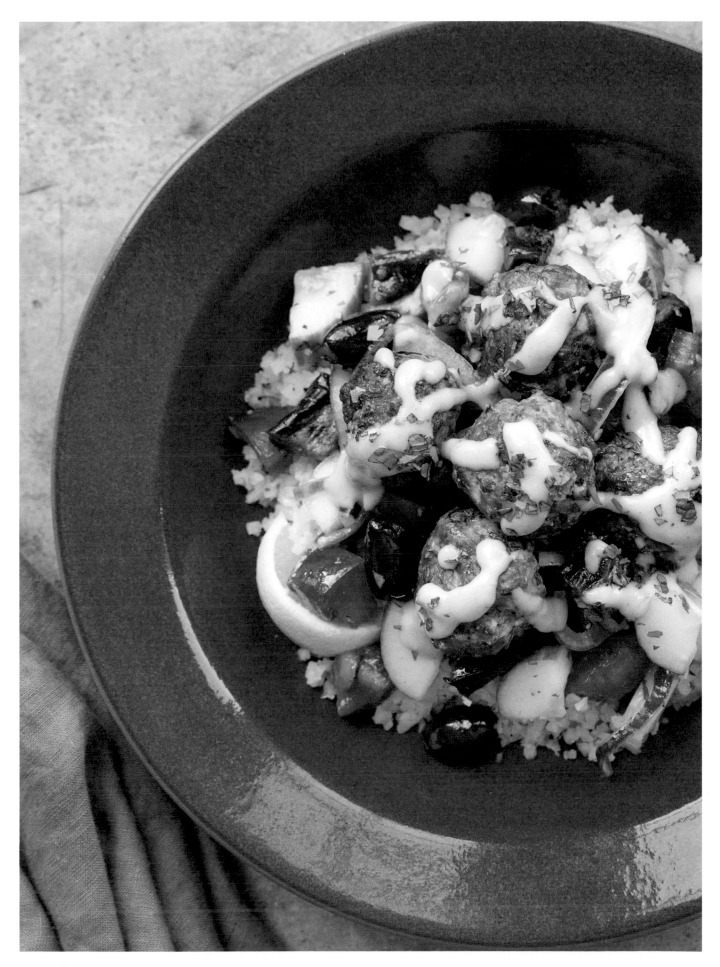

Grilled Pork Fall Salad

PREP TIME **20 MINUTES** • COOK TIME **15 MINUTES** • MAKES **2 SERVINGS**

NUTS

EGGS

NIGHTSHADES

FODMAPS

1 tablespoon cooking fat

2 (1-inch-thick) bone-in pork chops (6 to 8 ounces each)

1/2 tablespoon Smoky Spice Blend (page 248)

1/2 tablespoon Trifecta Spice Blend (page 249)

4 cups arugula

1 green apple, sliced into half moons

2 tablespoons Smoky Toasted Almonds (page 212)

2 tablespoons crumbled blue cheese or goat cheese (optional; Levels 1 & 2 only)

1/2 cup Balsamic Vinaigrette Dressing (page 238)

Preheat the oven to 400°F if you'll be using a grill pan or want to finish the chops in the oven.

Preheat a grill or grill pan to medium-high heat, then brush with the cooking fat. Season the pork chops liberally on both sides with the spice blends, then cook on the hot grill for 3 minutes per side, or until grill marks appear. (If the pork chops are less than an inch thick, cook for 2 minutes per side.)

If using a grill pan, transfer the pan to the oven and continue cooking for 4 to 8 minutes, until the chops reach an internal temperature of 145°F.

If using a grill, move the chops to a higher rack or lower-temperature area of the grill and cook until they're cooked through, about 3 to 5 minutes. Alternatively, you can transfer the chops from the grill to an oven-safe pan and bake them to finish cooking, following the instructions above for the grill pan.

Place the arugula in a large serving bowl and top with the pork chop, apple slices, almonds, and cheese, if using. Toss or top with the dressing before serving.

21DSD FRUIT SERVING

Each serving includes one half of a green apple. Factor this into your total intake of allowed fruit for the day.

NUT-FREE?

Omit the almonds or use sunflower or pumpkin seeds in their place.

LOW-FODMAP?

Swap in some raw carrots for the apple slices for some crunch. ●

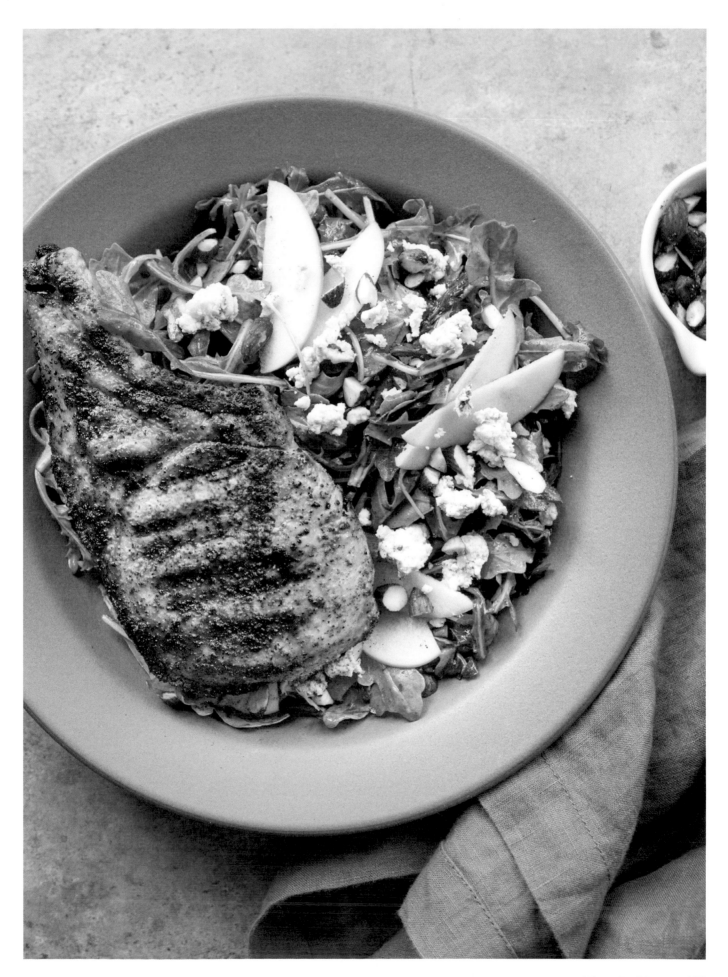

Super Garlic Meatballs with Fried Rice

PREP TIME **15 MINUTES** • COOK TIME **35 TO 45 MINUTES** •
MAKES **16 MEATBALLS (4 TO 6 PER SERVING)**

NUTS

EGGS

NIGHTSHADES

FODMAPS

1 pound ground pork

2 tablespoons Super Garlic Spice Blend (page 249)

FOR THE SAUCE

3/4 cup coconut aminos

1/2 teaspoon granulated garlic

1/4 teaspoon granulated onion

2 to 3 dashes of fish sauce

2 pinches of ginger powder

Sliced green onions, for garnish

1/2 batch Simple Fried Rice (page 192), for serving

Preheat the oven to 375°F. Line a rimmed baking sheet with foil and set a wire baking rack on it.

In a large mixing bowl, combine the pork and spice blend and mix well with your hands. Form the meat into sixteen 1-ounce meatballs (about the size of a golf ball) and place on the baking rack. Bake for 25 to 30 minutes, until slightly browned on the outside and cooked through so that no pink remains (you may want to cut into one to check for doneness).

While the meatballs cook, make the sauce: In a small saucepan, whisk together the ingredients for the sauce. Bring to a simmer over medium-low heat, then continue to simmer until the sauce reduces by half, 10 to 15 minutes. Tilt the pan frequently to prevent the sauce from burning.

Remove the meatballs from the oven and toss them in the sauce while they are still warm. Garnish with green onions and serve with fried rice.

NIGHTSHADE-FREE?
Omit the bell peppers from the fried rice recipe. ●

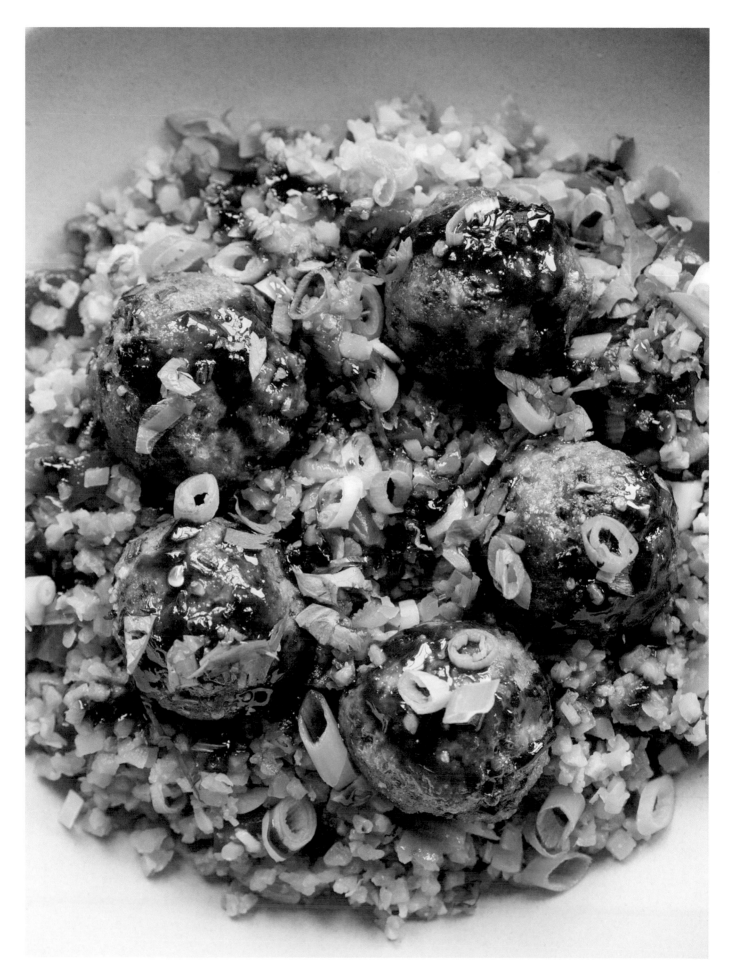

Sausage & Spinach "Polenta" Bowl

PREP TIME 5 MINUTES, PLUS 50 MINUTES FOR POLENTA AND 40 MINUTES FOR MARINARA • COOK TIME 10 MINUTES • MAKES 2 SERVINGS

NUTS

EGGS

NIGHTSHADES

FODMAPS

1 pound ground pork or other higher-fat ground meat of choice (see Note)

2 tablespoons Italian Spice Blend (page 248)

2 packed cups fresh spinach

2 cups Roasted Garlic Cauliflower Polenta (page 204)

1/2 cup grated Parmesan cheese (Levels 1 & 2 only)

1 cup Simple Marinara (page 237)

4 to 6 fresh basil leaves, for garnish (optional)

Heat a large skillet over medium heat. Combine the meat and spice blend in the skillet and cook for 5 minutes, breaking it up with a spatula as it cooks. Add the spinach and continue cooking for another 4 to 5 minutes, until the spinach begins to wilt and the meat is cooked through.

While the sausage is cooking, warm the cauliflower polenta in a small saucepan over medium heat. If using cheese, stir it into the cauliflower polenta.

At the same time, in a separate small saucepan, warm the marinara sauce over medium heat.

Remove the skillet with the sausage-and-spinach mixture from the heat. Divide the mixture in two and store one half in an airtight container in the refrigerator for up to 5 days.

Assemble the bowl: Divide the warmed cauliflower polenta between two serving bowls. Top each bowl with equal amounts of the sausage-and-spinach mixture and marinara sauce, and garnish with fresh basil leaves.

NOTE
If you're not using ground pork, you may want to add 2 tablespoons of your preferred cooking fat to the skillet.

KITCHEN TIP
Buy a premade 21DSD-friendly marinara sauce to help this meal come together quickly!

CHANGE IT UP
Add a poached egg for a satisfying breakfast bowl.
Mix things up by using kale instead of spinach. ●

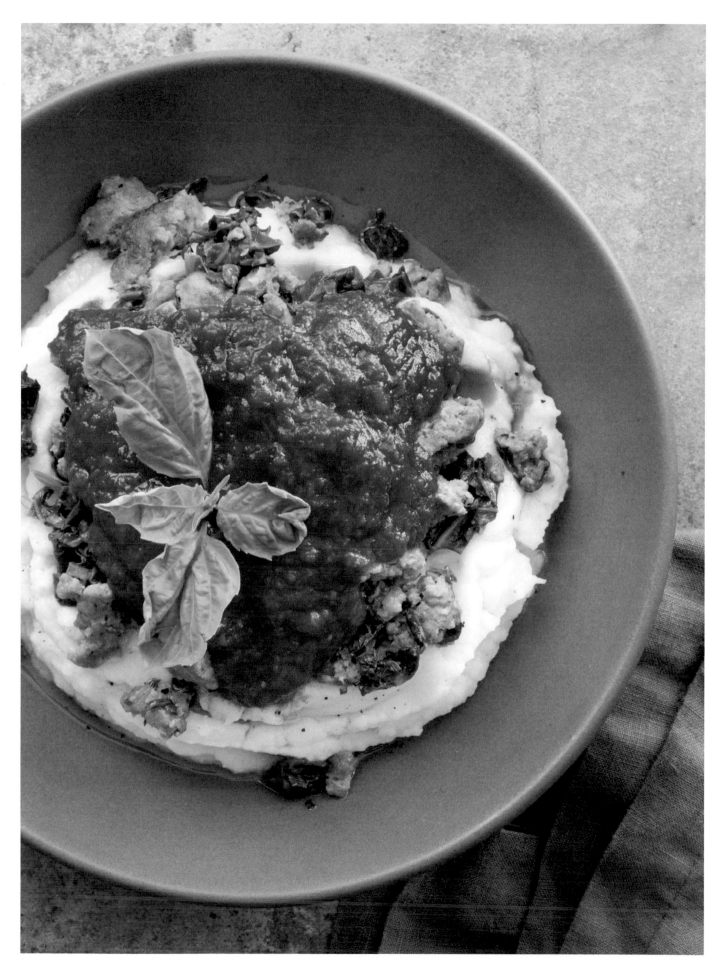

Super Garlic Salmon & Vegetables

PREP TIME **5 MINUTES** • COOK TIME **15 TO 20 MINUTES** • MAKES **2 SERVINGS**

NUTS

EGGS

NIGHTSHADES

FODMAPS

2 (6-ounce) fillets wild salmon

2 tablespoons melted ghee

Pinch of sea salt

Pinch of Super Garlic Spice Blend (page 249)

1 pound slender asparagus (about 1 bunch) or green beans, trimmed

1 lemon, plus more slices for garnish (optional)

Preheat the oven to 375°F.

Pat the salmon pieces dry with a paper towel to help remove any excess liquid. Brush the skin side with half the ghee and season with the salt. Flip the salmon over and brush with the remaining ghee and season with the spice blend. Place the salmon skin side down on a large baking sheet.

Spread the asparagus out in an even layer around the salmon pieces. If the asparagus seems too crowded, use a second baking sheet.

Cut the lemon in half and squeeze one half over the salmon and asparagus. Reserve the other half.

Bake for 12 to 15 minutes, until the salmon is cooked to your liking.

Squeeze the reserved lemon half over the top of the salmon and garnish with lemon slices, if desired, before serving.

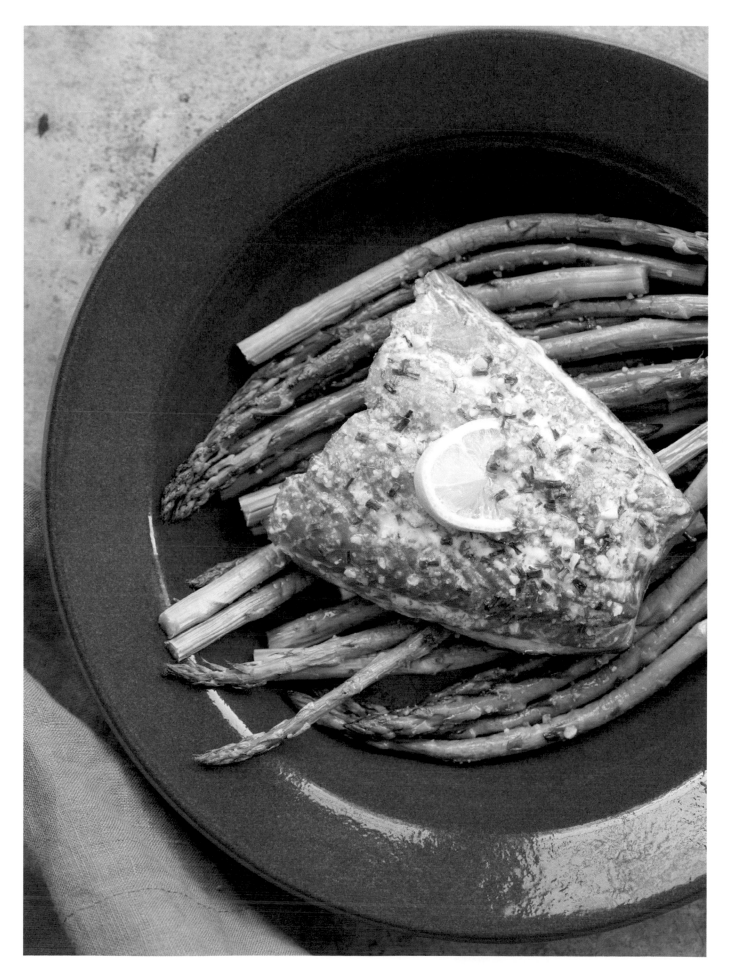

SNACKS & SIDES

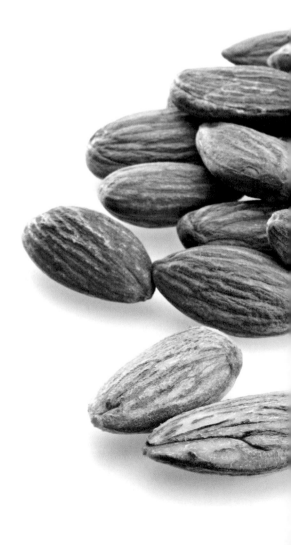

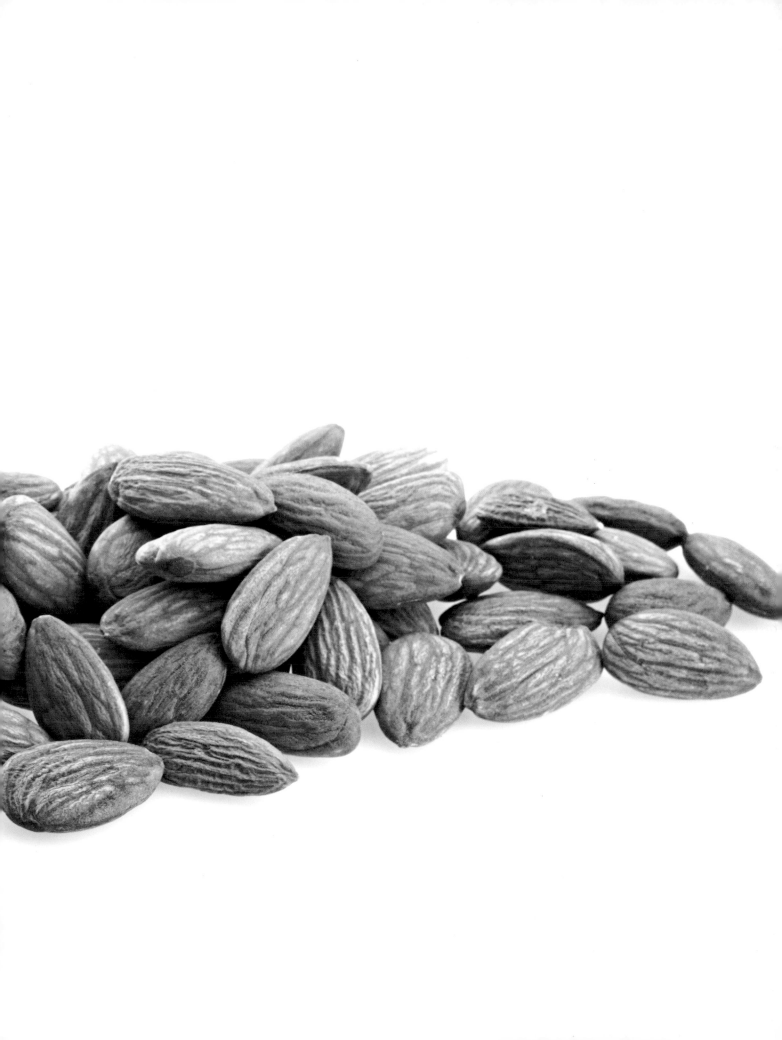

Simple Fried Rice

PREP TIME **10 MINUTES** • COOK TIME **15 TO 20 MINUTES** • MAKES **4 SERVINGS**

NUTS

EGGS

NIGHTSHADES

FODMAPS

1 tablespoon cooking fat

1 medium red onion, diced

1 red bell pepper, diced

Few pinches of sea salt

4 cloves garlic, grated or minced

2 (12-ounce) packages riced cauliflower (see page 127)

1/4 cup coconut aminos

2 teaspoons sesame oil

Few dashes of fish sauce

Few pinches of ginger powder

1/4 cup chopped fresh cilantro

1/4 cup sliced green onions, plus more for garnish

Heat the cooking fat in a large skillet over medium heat. Add the onion, bell pepper, and salt to the skillet and cook for 8 to 10 minutes, until the onions start to turn translucent and the peppers start to lose their crunch. Add the garlic and cook for 1 to 2 minutes more, until the garlic starts to turn golden brown.

Add the riced cauliflower, coconut aminos, sesame oil, fish sauce, and ginger powder and stir to combine. Cook for 5 to 8 minutes, until the cauliflower is soft but not mushy.

Remove from heat and mix in the cilantro and green onions, or mix them in at the very end of cooking to leave them as fresh as uncooked. Serve garnished with additional green onions.

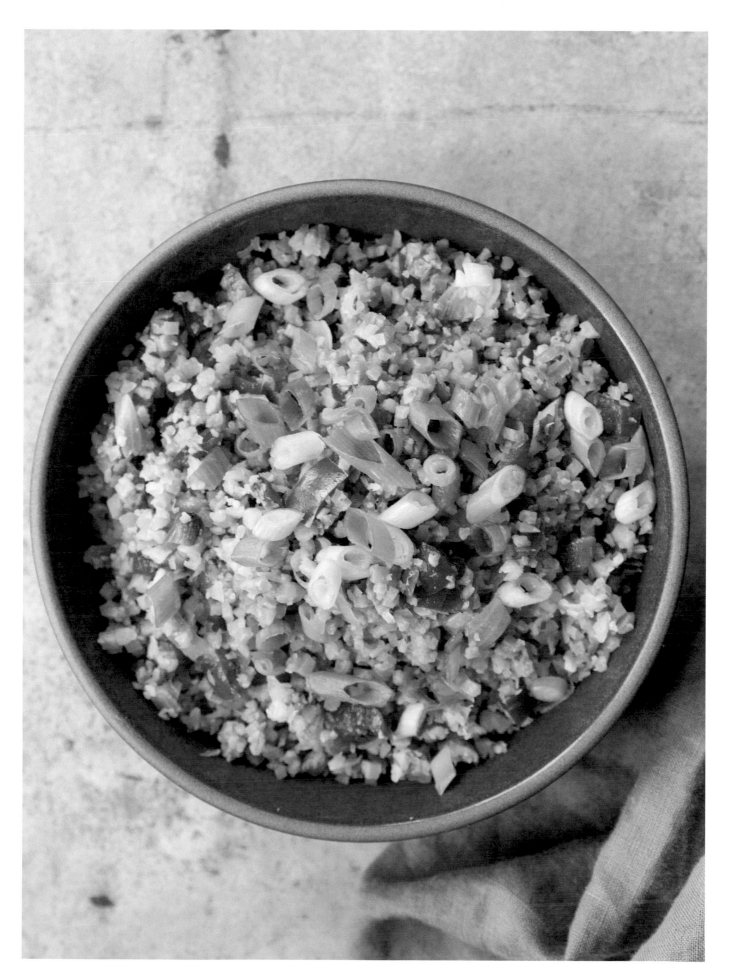

Crispy Brussels Sprouts

PREP TIME **10 MINUTES** • COOK TIME **25 TO 30 MINUTES** •
MAKES **2 SERVINGS (ABOUT 1 CUP EACH)**

NUTS

EGGS

NIGHTSHADES

FODMAPS

4 cups Brussels sprouts
(about 1 pound), trimmed
and halved

1 tablespoon cooking fat

1 teaspoon Trifecta Spice
Blend (page 249)

Preheat the oven to 375°F.

Place the Brussels sprouts on a large rimmed
baking sheet (use stainless steel rather than
nonstick for the best browning). Toss with the
cooking fat.

Sprinkle with the spice blend, then arrange cut side
down.

Roast for 25 to 30 minutes, until the leaves begin
to separate and become dark brown and crispy and
the halves are cooked through and browned. Check
about halfway through cooking—if the separated
leaves have browned very quickly, remove them,
then continue roasting the rest of the pieces.

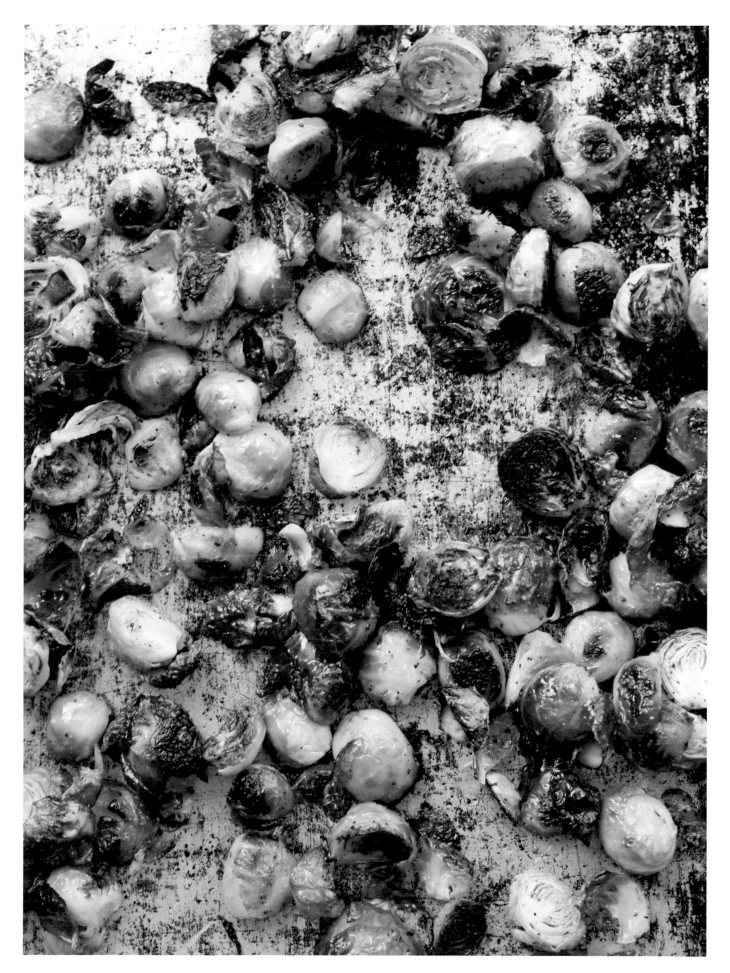

Garlic Butter Sautéed Mushrooms

PREP TIME **10 MINUTES** • COOK TIME **15 TO 20 MINUTES** • MAKES **2 SERVINGS**

NUTS
EGGS
NIGHTSHADES
FODMAPS

3 to 4 tablespoons butter or ghee

4 cloves garlic, minced or grated

1 pound mushrooms (any kind), sliced

Pinch of sea salt

Pinch of ground black pepper

Chopped fresh chives, for garnish (optional)

In a large skillet, melt the butter or ghee over medium-high heat. Add the garlic and stir for 30 seconds.

Add the mushrooms, salt, and pepper and stir to coat. Let sit for 2 to 3 minutes, stir again, and then cook for 10 to 15 more minutes, until fork-tender. Taste for seasoning and add more salt and pepper if necessary. Garnish with chives, if desired.

Store in an airtight container in the fridge for up to 5 days.

KITCHEN TIP
Use presliced mushrooms to save time! ●

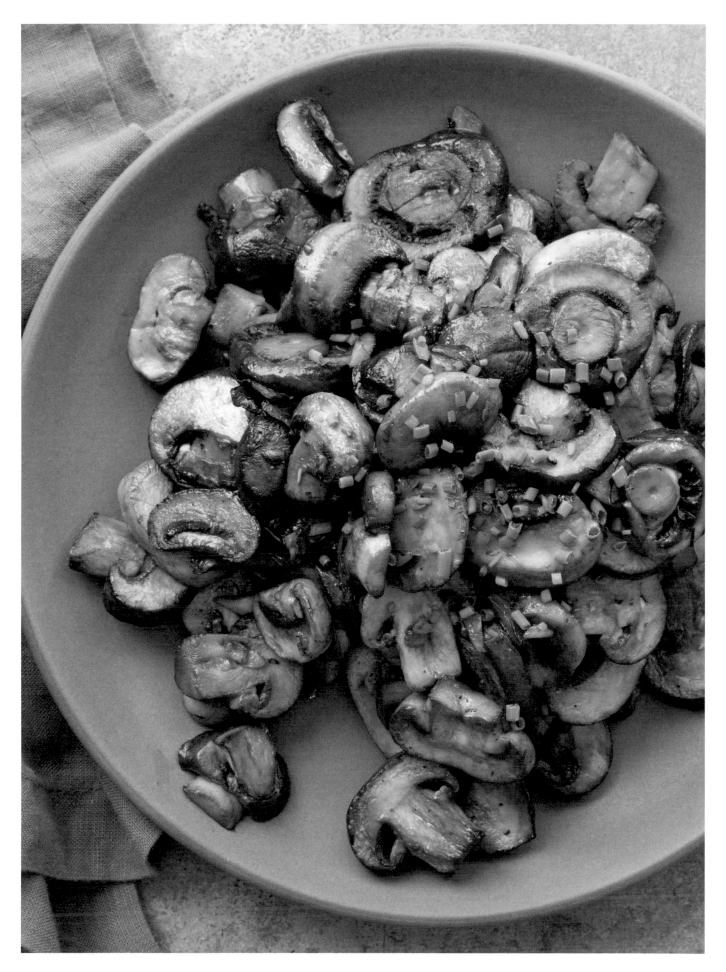

Pesto Roasted Carrots

PREP TIME **5 MINUTES** • COOK TIME **25 TO 30 MINUTES** • MAKES **2 SERVINGS**

NUTS

EGGS

NIGHTSHADES

FODMAPS

8 medium carrots, halved lengthwise

2 tablespoons cooking fat

Sea salt and ground black pepper

1/4 cup Pesto Sauce (page 236)

Preheat the oven to 375°F.

Place the carrots on a large rimmed baking sheet, toss with the cooking fat, and sprinkle with salt and pepper.

Spread the carrots in an even layer and roast for 25 to 30 minutes, until fork-tender and browned and slightly crispy around the edges.

Drizzle with the pesto sauce and serve.

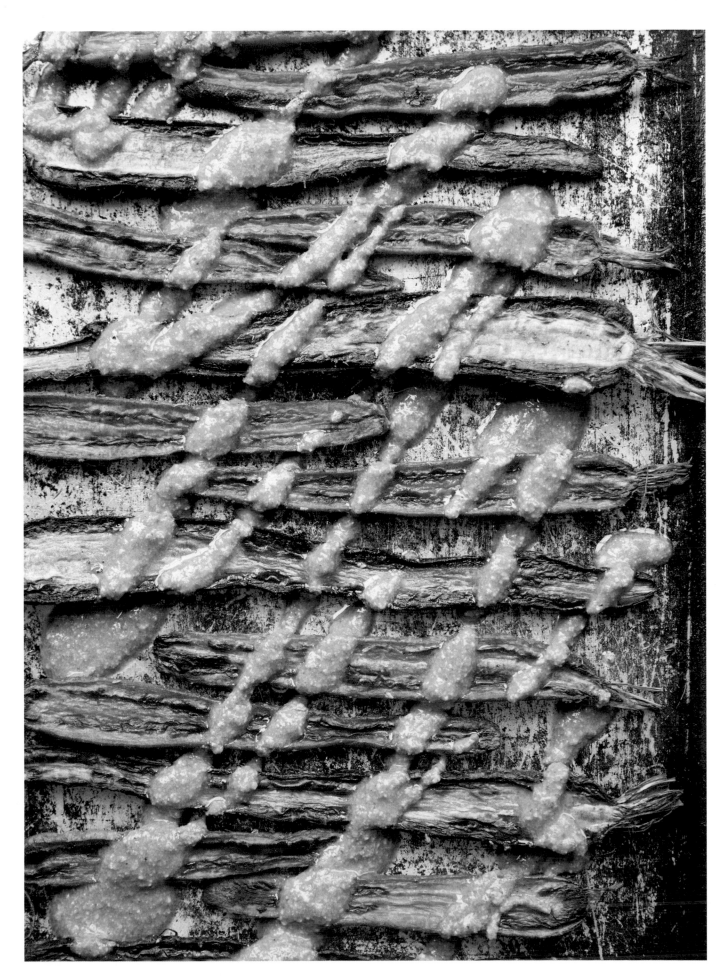

Crispy Broccoli

PREP TIME **10 MINUTES** • COOK TIME **20 TO 30 MINUTES** •
MAKES **2 SERVINGS (ABOUT 1 CUP PER SERVING)**

NUTS
EGGS
NIGHTSHADES
FODMAPS

1 large head broccoli, cut into florets

1 tablespoon cooking fat

1 teaspoon Trifecta Spice Blend (page 249)

A few pinches of red pepper flakes

Juice of 1/2 fresh lemon

Preheat the oven to 375°F.

Place the broccoli florets on a large rimmed baking sheet (preferably stainless steel rather than nonstick for the best browning). Toss them with the cooking fat and spice blend.

Roast for 20 to 30 minutes, until the broccoli ends become dark brown and crispy. Sprinkle with the red pepper flakes and lemon juice before serving.

NIGHTSHADE-FREE?
Omit the red pepper flakes.

KITCHEN TIP
Buy your broccoli pre-cut into florets to save time! ●

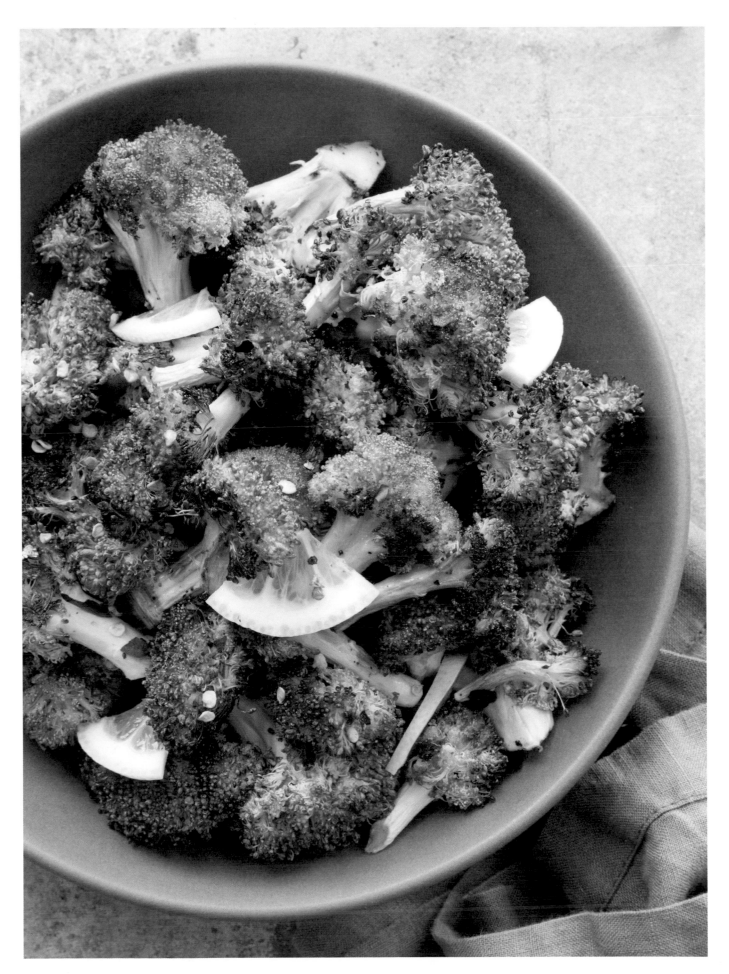

Roasted Butternut Squash

PREP TIME **10 MINUTES** • COOK TIME **30 TO 40 MINUTES** • MAKES **2 SERVINGS**

NUTS

EGGS

NIGHTSHADES

FODMAPS

1 large butternut squash (2 to 3 pounds), peeled and cut into 1-inch cubes

2 tablespoons cooking fat

1 1/2 teaspoons Trifecta Spice Blend (page 249)

A few pinches of ground cinnamon (optional)

Preheat the oven to 375°F.

Place the cubed butternut squash on a large rimmed baking sheet (preferably stainless steel rather than nonstick for the best browning). Toss with the cooking fat and sprinkle with the spices, then spread evenly on the baking sheet.

Roast for 30 to 40 minutes, until the edges start to crisp and the squash is cooked through and browned.

KITCHEN TIP
Buy pre-cut butternut squash in bags in the refrigerated section of your grocery store to save time! ●

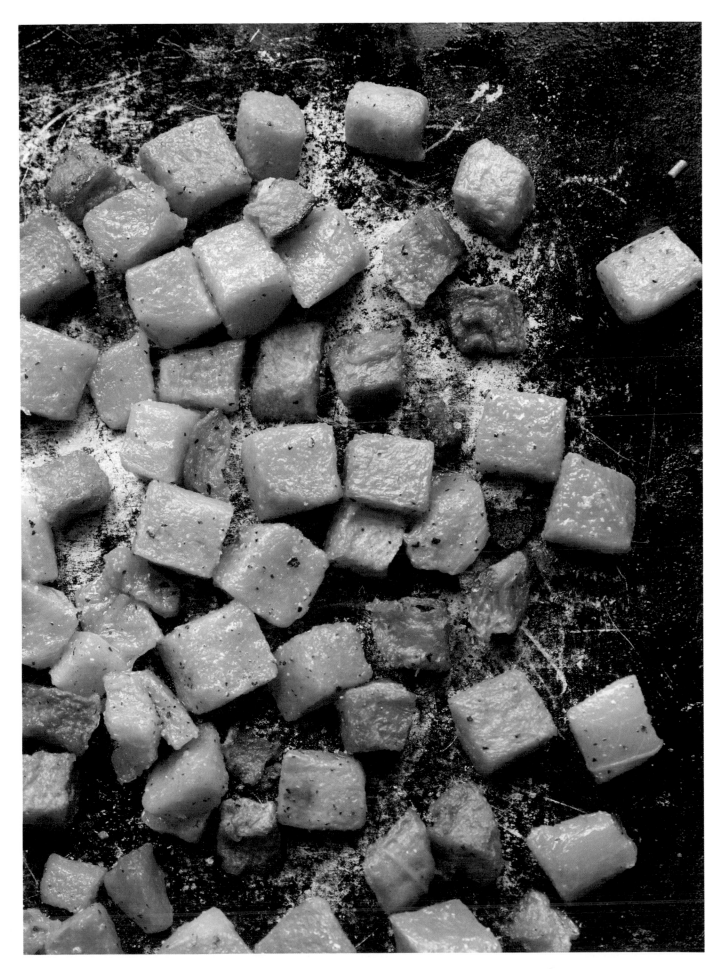

Roasted Garlic Cauliflower Polenta

PREP TIME **15 MINUTES** • COOK TIME **45 MINUTES** •
MAKES **2 TO 3 CUPS (1 CUP PER SERVING)**

NUTS
EGGS
NIGHTSHADES
FODMAPS

1 head garlic

4 tablespoons cooking fat, divided

2 small heads or 1 large head cauliflower, roughly chopped into 2- to 3-inch pieces

Sea salt and ground black pepper

Melted ghee, for drizzling

KITCHEN TIP
If you don't have a food processor, you can use a high-powered blender like a Vitamix or Blendtec, or mash the steamed cauliflower by hand with a potato masher.

TIME-SAVING TIP
Make this with 2 to 3 teaspoons of garlic powder instead of roasted garlic if you want to save time, but know that the flavor will not be as rich and amazing. ●

Preheat the oven to 350°F.

Slice the tips off of the head of garlic, then place it cut side up on a large square of foil. Top with 2 tablespoons of the cooking fat and wrap the foil around the garlic.

Roast for about 45 minutes, until the skin is darker in color and cloves are golden brown and soft. When the garlic is done and cool enough to handle, gently squeeze each clove out of the skin.

While the garlic roasts, steam the cauliflower: Place the cauliflower pieces in a steamer basket over 2 inches of water, or in a large pot with about 2 inches of water, on medium-high heat. Steam until fork-tender, about 15 minutes.

Place the steamed cauliflower in a food processor and add the remaining 2 tablespoons of cooking fat, the roasted garlic cloves, and a few pinches of salt and pepper. Puree until smooth and creamy. Taste and adjust the seasoning as needed. Drizzle with melted ghee, if desired.

Store leftovers in an airtight container in the fridge for up to 5 days.

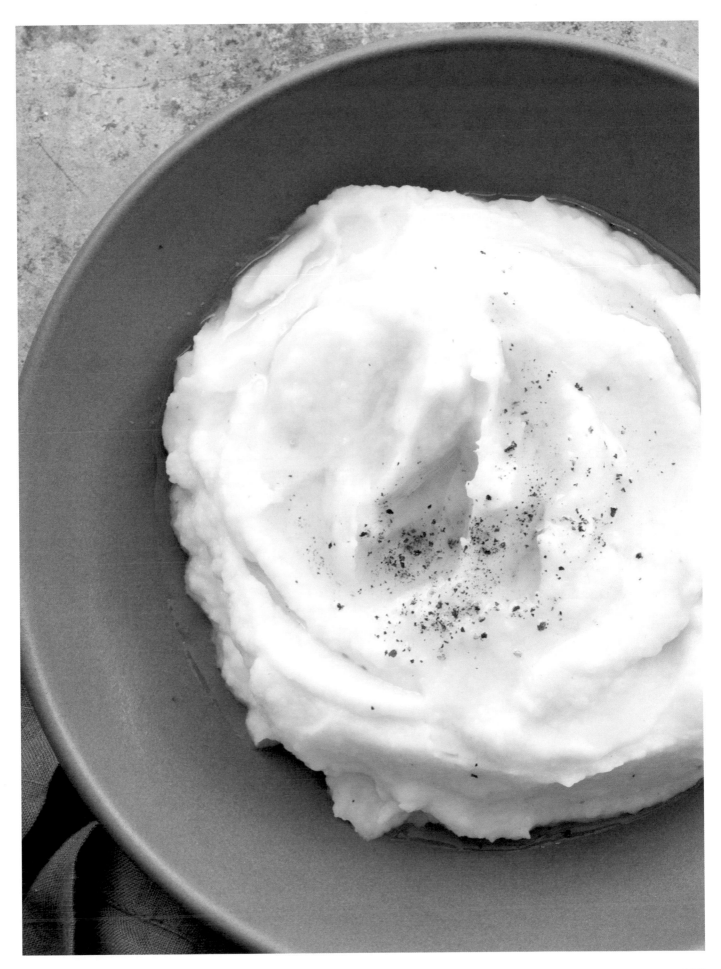

Ranch Roasted Potatoes

PREP TIME **10 MINUTES** • COOK TIME **45 TO 55 MINUTES** • MAKES **4 SERVINGS**

NUTS

EGGS

NIGHTSHADES

FODMAPS

1 pound yellow or red potatoes, chopped into 1-inch pieces

2 tablespoons cooking fat

2 tablespoons Ranch Spice Blend (page 249)

Preheat the oven to 375°F.

In a large mixing bowl, combine the potatoes, cooking fat, and spice blend and toss until the potatoes are well coated.

Transfer the potatoes to a 9 by 13-inch baking pan and spread out into an even layer.

Roast in the oven for 45 to 55 minutes, until brown and crispy, tossing halfway through.

Store leftovers in an airtight container in the refrigerator for up to 5 days. To reheat, place in an oven or toaster oven at 350°F for 10 minutes.

NIGHTSHADE-FREE?
Use sweet potatoes instead of white potatoes. ●

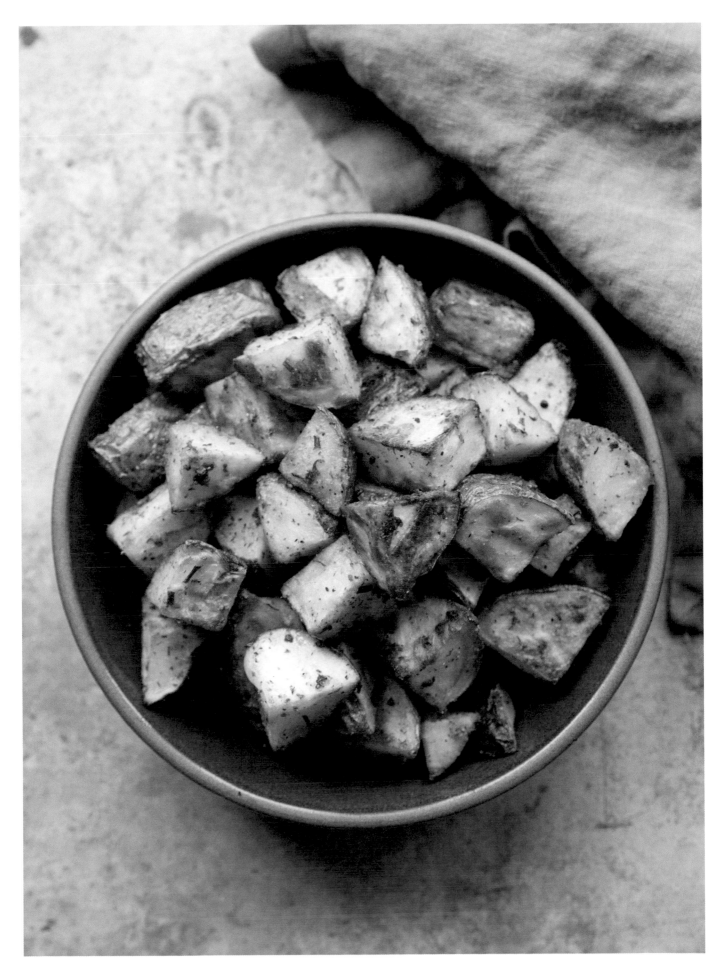

Roasted Eggplant Steaks with Tahini Sauce

PREP TIME **15 MINUTES** • COOK TIME **40 MINUTES** • MAKES **2 SERVINGS**

NUTS
EGGS
NIGHTSHADES
FODMAPS

1 large eggplant, cut into 1/2-inch slices

3 tablespoons extra-virgin olive oil

Sea salt and ground black pepper

FOR THE TAHINI SAUCE

1/2 cup tahini

Juice of 1 fresh lemon

2 tablespoons extra-virgin olive oil

2 tablespoons water

1/4 teaspoon sea salt

1 to 2 large cloves garlic, peeled

FOR SERVING

1/2 fresh lemon

2 tablespoons toasted pine nuts

A few pinches of paprika

1/4 cup chopped fresh cilantro

Preheat the oven to 350°F.

Brush both sides of the eggplant slices with the olive oil (or use your hands to massage it into the eggplant) and season both sides with a few pinches of salt and pepper. Bake for 20 minutes, flip the eggplant slices, then bake for 20 minutes more, until the eggplant is browned and the flesh is softened and darker in color all the way through.

While the eggplant is baking, make the tahini sauce: Combine all the sauce ingredients except the garlic in a blender and blend until smooth. Add 1 large clove of garlic, blend until smooth, then taste and add another clove if desired. Note that raw garlic will intensify in flavor over time, so be careful not to overdo it initially.

To serve, drizzle the eggplant with the tahini sauce and garnish with a squeeze of fresh lemon juice, toasted pine nuts, paprika, and chopped cilantro.

KITCHEN TIP
To thin the tahini sauce and make it into a salad dressing, add 2 more tablespoons of water and 2 more tablespoons of olive oil when blending.

NUT-FREE?
Omit the pine nuts.

FODMAP-FREE?
Omit the garlic. ●

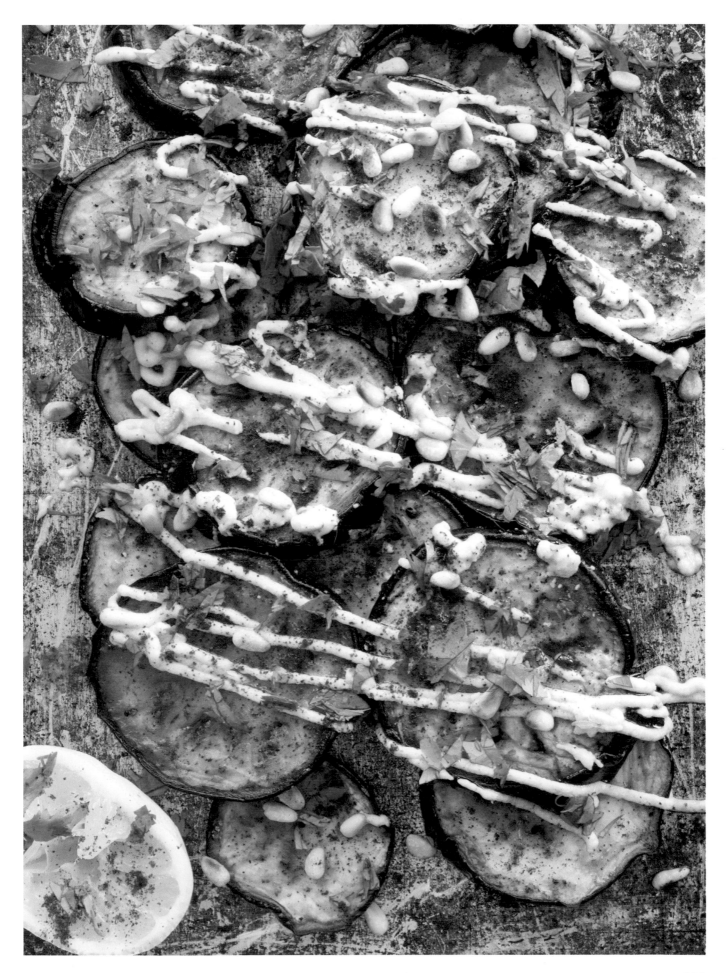

Simple Deviled Eggs

PREP TIME **10 MINUTES** • COOK TIME **20 MINUTES** •
MAKES **4 SERVINGS (4 EGG HALVES PER SERVING)**

NUTS

EGGS

NIGHTSHADES

FODMAPS

8 eggs

1/3 cup mayonnaise, store-bought or homemade (page 246)

1 teaspoon gluten-free Dijon mustard

Smoky Spice Blend (page 248) or Everything Bagel Spice Blend (page 248), for garnish

Chopped fresh chives, for garnish (optional)

Fill a medium-sized pot with water and bring to a boil over high heat (about 10 minutes). Gently lower the eggs into the water and boil with the lid off for 10 minutes.

While the eggs boil, fill a large bowl with cold water and ice. After the eggs have boiled for 10 minutes, place them gently into the ice bath for 5 minutes.

Cut each hard-boiled egg in half lengthwise and place the yolks in a medium-sized mixing bowl with the mayonnaise and mustard. Mix until creamy and completely combined.

Spoon the yolk-mayonnaise mixture evenly into the egg white halves and sprinkle the spice blend over the finished eggs. Garnish with chives, if desired.

Store leftovers in an airtight container in the fridge for up to 3 days.

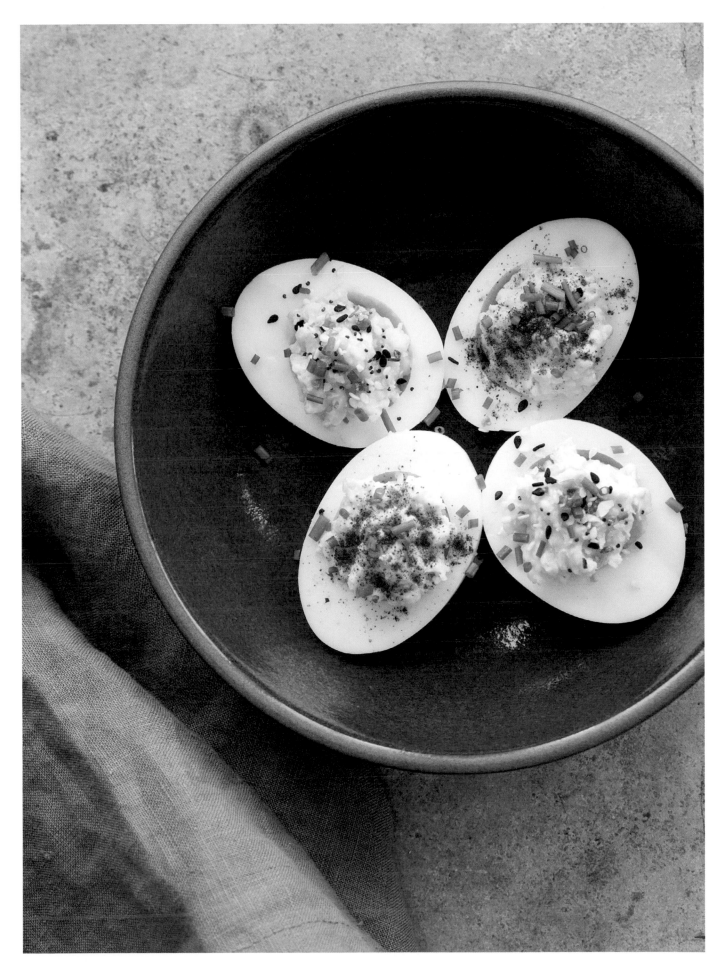

Smoky Toasted Nut Mix

PREP TIME — • COOK TIME **5 MINUTES** • MAKES **4 SERVINGS**

NUTS

EGGS

NIGHTSHADES

FODMAPS

1 tablespoon extra-virgin olive oil

1 cup raw nuts, such as cashews, almonds, or walnuts, or a combination

1 tablespoon Smoky Spice Blend (page 248)

In a small skillet, warm the olive oil over medium-low heat.

Add the almonds and spice blend and stir to combine. Cook for approximately 4 to 5 minutes, until browned and fragrant, stirring constantly.

Store in an airtight container at room temperature for up to a week or in the refrigerator for up to 3 weeks.

VARIATION: SMOKY TOASTED ALMONDS
Instead of mixed nuts, use 1 cup raw almonds. ●

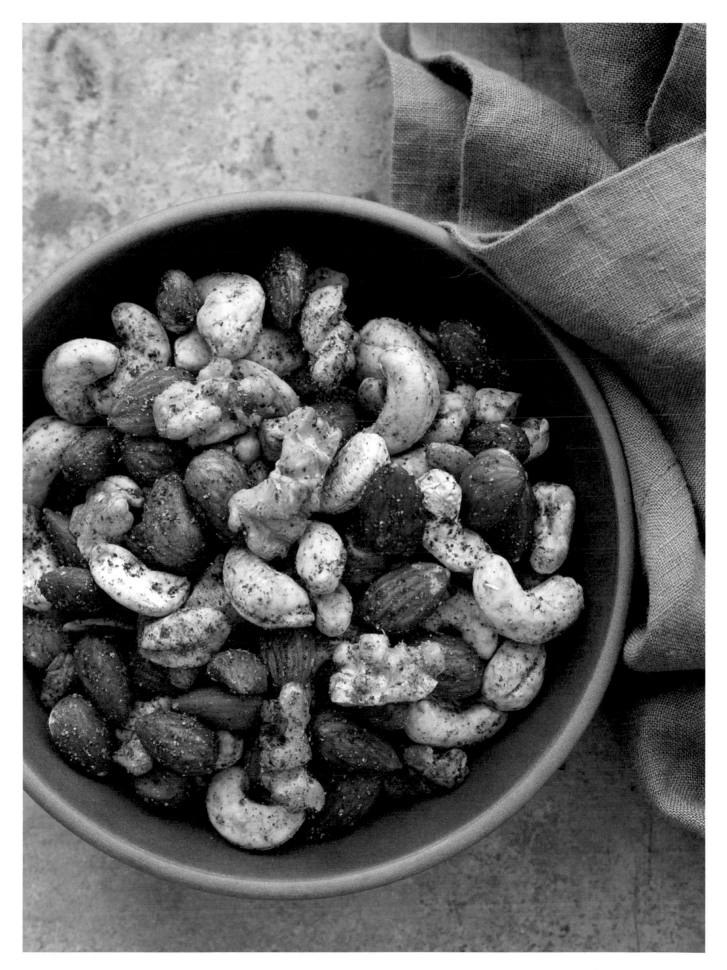

Cinnilla Nut Mix

PREP TIME **5 MINUTES** • COOK TIME **25 TO 30 MINUTES** • MAKES **4 SERVINGS**

NUTS

EGGS

NIGHTSHADES

FODMAPS

1 egg white

1 tablespoon coconut oil, melted

1/4 teaspoon pure vanilla extract

1 teaspoon ground cinnamon

2 pinches of sea salt

1/2 cup walnuts

1/4 cup almonds

1/4 cup macadamia nuts

2 tablespoons almond meal, store-bought or homemade (page 242)

Preheat the oven to 275°F.

In a mixing bowl, whisk together the egg white, coconut oil, vanilla, cinnamon, and salt. Add the nuts (you may substitute others of your choice) and almond meal, and toss to evenly coat.

Spread the nuts evenly on a rimmed baking sheet and bake for 25 to 30 minutes, until toasted.

Spicy Thai Nut Mix

PREP TIME **5 MINUTES** • COOK TIME **25 TO 30 MINUTES** • MAKES **4 SERVINGS**

NUTS

EGGS

NIGHTSHADES

FODMAPS

1 tablespoon coconut aminos

1 tablespoon coconut oil, melted

2 to 4 drops fish sauce

Zest and juice of 1 lime

1/4 teaspoon cayenne pepper

1/8 teaspoon minced fresh ginger, or more to taste

1/4 cup almonds

1/4 cup pepitas (pumpkin seeds)

1/2 cup walnuts

1 teaspoon sesame seeds

Preheat the oven to 275°F.

In a medium-sized mixing bowl, whisk together the coconut aminos, coconut oil, fish sauce, lime zest, lime juice, cayenne pepper, and ginger. Add the nuts and seeds (you may substitute others of your choice) and toss to evenly coat.

Spread the nuts evenly on a baking sheet and bake for 25 to 30 minutes, until toasted.

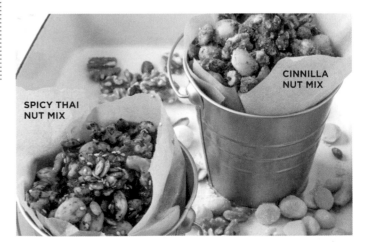

CINNILLA
NUT MIX

SPICY THAI
NUT MIX

Simple Beef Jerky

PREP TIME **5 MINUTES, PLUS 1 HOUR TO MARINATE** • COOK TIME **2 TO 4 HOURS IN THE OVEN OR 3 TO 5 HOURS IN A DEHYDRATOR** • MAKES **4 TO 6 SERVINGS**

FOR THE MARINADE

1/3 cup coconut aminos

1 teaspoon granulated garlic

1 teaspoon onion powder

1/2 teaspoon sea salt

1/4 teaspoon ground black pepper

1 pound lean beef (London broil or a roast with the fat trimmed works well), chicken, or turkey

In a large bowl, whisk together the marinade ingredients. Taste and adjust the seasonings as desired; it should taste stronger than you want the finished jerky to taste.

Cutting against the grain of the meat, slice the meat thinly into approximately 1/8-inch-thick slices using a very sharp knife or a meat slicer.

Place the sliced meat in the marinade, cover, and marinate at room temperature or in the refrigerator for up to 1 hour.

To use a food dehydrator: Arrange the meat on the trays of the dehydrator and heat at 135°F to 145°F until the meat reaches the desired dryness. This should take approximately 3 to 5 hours.

To use the oven: Preheat to 200°F. Bake for 2 to 4 hours, until the jerky reaches the desired level of dryness.

NUTS

EGGS

NIGHTSHADES

FODMAPS

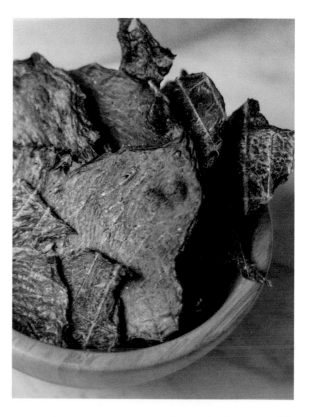

NOT-SWEET TREATS

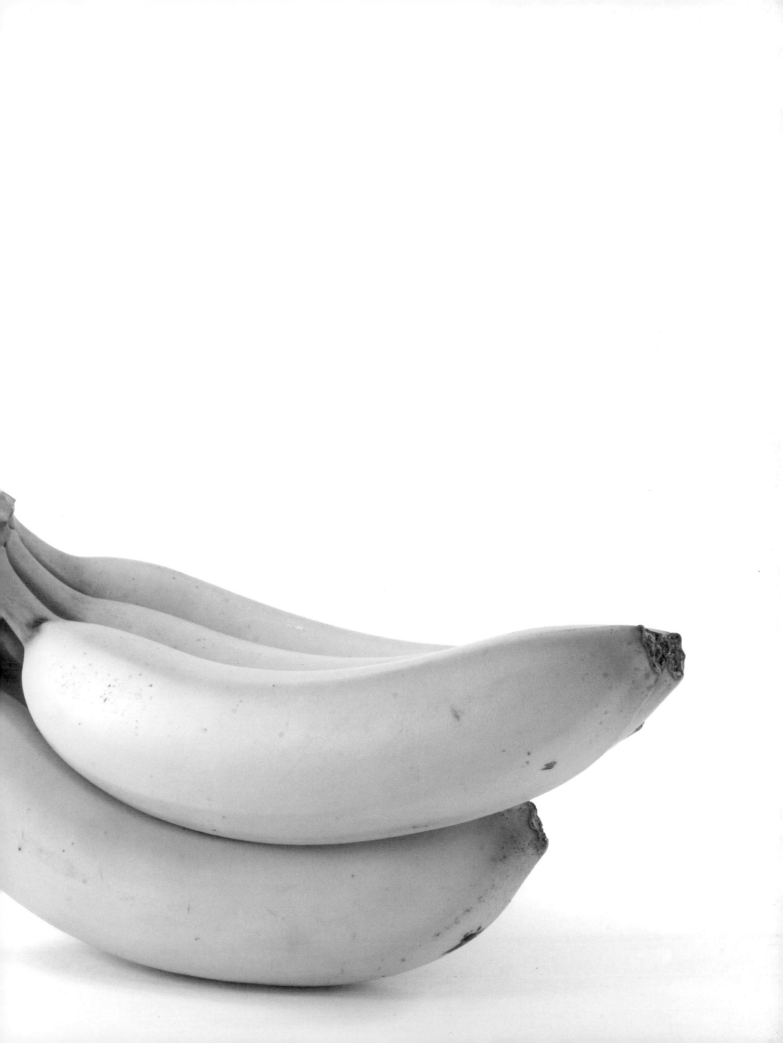

Two-Bite Chocolate Cream Pies

PREP TIME **15 MINUTES** • COOK TIME **10 MINUTES** •
MAKES **12 PIES (3 PIES PER SERVING)**

NUTS

EGGS

NIGHTSHADES

FODMAPS

FOR THE CRUST

1/2 cup chopped raw cashews or walnuts

1/2 cup unsweetened finely shredded coconut

1 tablespoon ghee, melted

2 pinches of sea salt

2 pinches of ground cinnamon

FOR THE MOO-LESS CHOCOLATE PUDDING

1 avocado, halved and pitted

1 medium green-tipped banana

1/4 cup full-fat coconut milk, store-bought or homemade (page 243)

2 tablespoons unsweetened cocoa powder

1 tablespoon unsweetened carob powder (see Note)

1/4 teaspoon pure vanilla extract

FOR GARNISH (OPTIONAL)

1 tablespoon cacao nibs

1 tablespoon toasted coconut flakes

SPECIAL EQUIPMENT

1 (12-cavity) mini-muffin tin

12 parchment paper mini baking cups

Preheat the oven to 350°F. Line a 12-cavity mini-muffin tin with parchment paper mini baking cups.

Make the crust: Place the chopped cashews, shredded coconut, ghee, salt, and cinnamon in a food processor. Pulse until the texture is fine and the ingredients are well combined.

Press the crust into the prepared muffin tin and bake for 10 minutes, or until lightly browned and starting to crisp. Set aside to cool.

While the crust is baking, make the Moo-Less Chocolate Pudding: Scoop the flesh of the avocado into a food processor and add the banana, coconut milk, cocoa powder, carob powder, and vanilla extract. Blend until completely smooth, scraping down the sides once or twice.

Fill the cooled crusts with the chocolate pudding. Garnish with cacao nibs and/or toasted coconut flakes, if desired. Serve at room temperature or chilled.

Store in an airtight container in the fridge for up to 3 days or in the freezer for up to 2 weeks. To defrost, allow to come to room temperature for about 15 to 20 minutes.

NOTE

If you can't find carob powder, use another tablespoon of cocoa powder instead (3 tablespoons total). But the carob powder will add a hint of sweetness without adding sweetener, so it's worth using if you can! ●

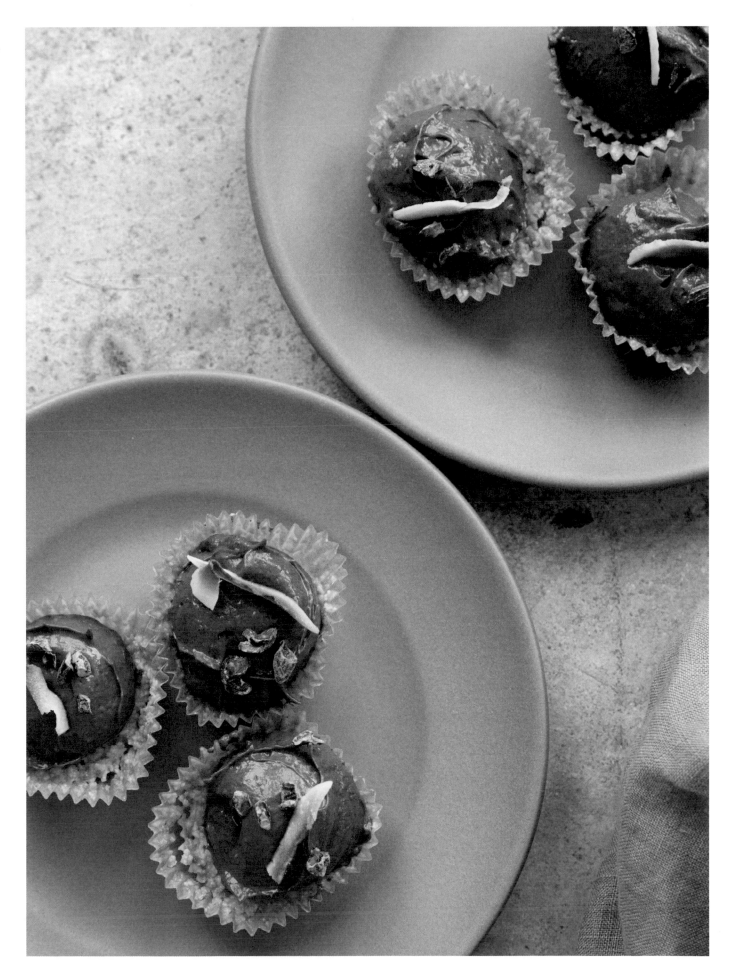

NOT-SWEET TREATS

21DSD Cinnamon Banana Bread

PREP TIME **5 MINUTES, PLUS 5 MINUTES TO CHILL THE BANANAS** •
COOK TIME **45 MINUTES** • MAKES **ONE 8 1/2 BY 4 1/2-INCH LOAF (8 TO 10 SLICES)**

NUTS
EGGS
NIGHTSHADES
FODMAPS

- 3 tablespoons coconut oil, divided
- 3 medium green-tipped bananas, diced
- 9 eggs
- 1 1/2 teaspoons pure vanilla extract
- 3/4 cup + 3 tablespoons full-fat coconut milk, store-bought or homemade (page 243)
- 1 1/2 teaspoons apple cider vinegar
- 1 cup cashew flour, sifted
- 3/4 cup coconut flour, sifted
- 3 teaspoons ground cinnamon
- 1 1/2 teaspoons baking soda
- 1/4 teaspoon sea salt
- Cacao nibs, for garnish (optional)

Preheat the oven to 350°F. Brush an 8 1/2 by 4 1/2-inch loaf pan with butter or ghee and line with parchment paper.

In a skillet over medium heat, melt 1 tablespoon of the coconut oil. Add the bananas and sauté until soft, approximately 8 to 10 minutes. Place the cooked bananas in the refrigerator to chill for at least 5 minutes.

In a large mixing bowl, vigorously whisk the eggs, vanilla, remaining 2 tablespoons of coconut oil, coconut milk, and vinegar for about 20 seconds, until combined. Add the cashew flour, coconut flour, cinnamon, baking soda, cooked and chilled bananas, and salt to the egg mixture and whisk vigorously until smooth.

Pour the batter into the prepared loaf pan, filling the pan about two-thirds full, as the bread will puff up while baking. Top with cacao nibs if desired.

Bake for 30 to 35 minutes, until the loaf is puffed-up and golden brown. Allow to cool completely before slicing.

Serve toasted or warm, either plain or with butter, ghee, or coconut butter and extra ground cinnamon on top.

Store leftovers in an airtight container on the counter for up to 3 days, in the refrigerator for up to a week, or in the freezer for up to 3 weeks. Slice and toast from the fridge or defrost on the countertop overnight and toast the following day.

VARIATION: BANANA NUT MUFFINS
Line a 12-cavity muffin tin with parchment paper baking cups. Pour the batter into the prepared tin, filling each cavity about two-thirds full (the muffins will puff up while baking). Top each muffin with a walnut half.

21DSD FRUIT SERVING
For a loaf, cut into 9 slices; each slice includes about one-third of a green-tipped banana. Factor this into your total intake of allowed fruit for the day.

KITCHEN TIP
You can use a parchment paper loaf pan liner for easy removal and slicing.

CHANGE IT UP
Make this a fall-flavored pumpkin bread by swapping 3/4 cup pumpkin purée for the banana and pumpkin pie spice for the ground cinnamon, and using 2 tablespoons of coconut oil instead of 3. ●

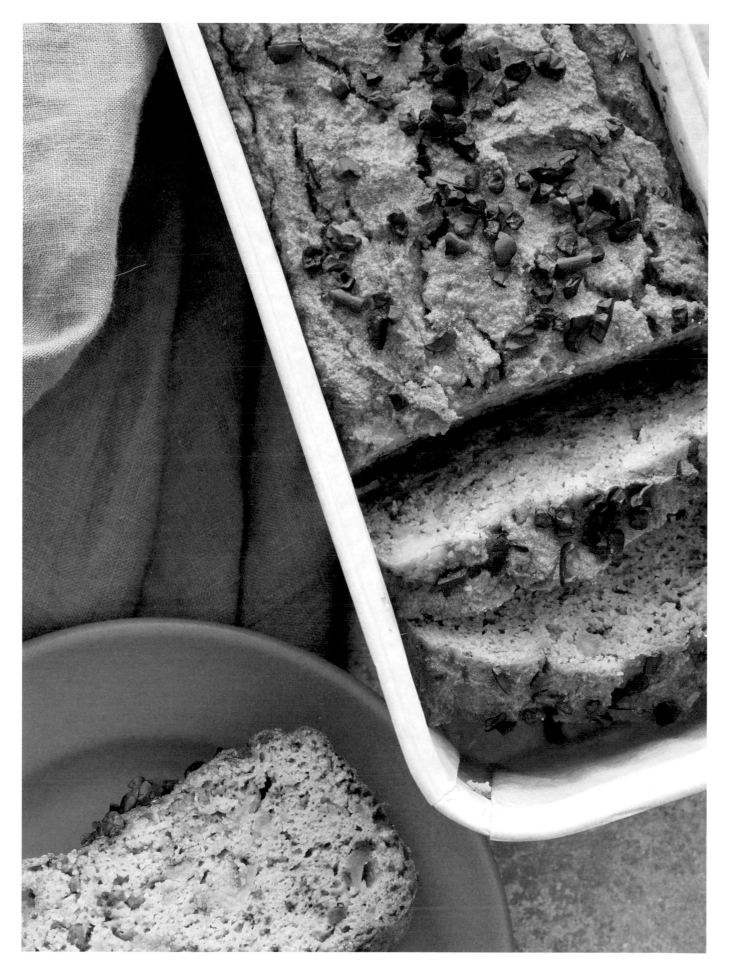

21DSD Frozen Coco-Monkey Bites

PREP TIME **5 MINUTES, PLUS AN HOUR TO CHILL** • COOK TIME **LESS THAN 5 MINUTES** • MAKES **6 SERVINGS**

NUTS
EGGS
NIGHTSHADES
FODMAPS

1/4 cup coconut oil

2 tablespoons peanut butter or other nut or seed butter

2 tablespoons unsweetened cocoa powder

2 tablespoons unsweetened carob powder (see Note)

1/4 teaspoon pure vanilla extract

Pinch of sea salt

3 medium green-tipped bananas, sliced into 1/2-inch coins

Unsweetened shredded coconut, for garnish (optional)

Cacao nibs, for garnish (optional)

Melt all the ingredients except the bananas in a double boiler over medium-high heat for just a few minutes. (If you don't have a double boiler, a heatproof glass mixing bowl set on top of a saucepan will also work.) Alternatively, place the ingredients in a small microwave-safe bowl and microwave on high in 20-second increments until smooth, stirring after each increment.

Place the mixture in the refrigerator and chill for 5 to 10 minutes, until slightly firm.

Dip each banana slice in the chilled chocolate mixture and set on a wire rack over a baking sheet. Garnish with coconut and cacao nibs, if using, and place in the refrigerator to set for about an hour.

Once set, transfer the bites evenly into six resealable plastic bags or freezer-safe containers—these are single-serving portions. Store in the freezer for up to several weeks and enjoy frozen.

NOTE
If you can't find carob powder, use 2 more tablespoons of cocoa powder instead (4 tablespoons total). But the carob powder will add a hint of sweetness without adding sweetener, so it's worth using if you can!

21DSD FRUIT SERVING
One serving includes half of a green-tipped banana. Factor this into your total intake of allowed fruit for the day. Limit yourself to one serving of this recipe per day.

NUT-FREE?
Make these with sunflower seed butter!

FODMAP-FREE?
Make these with ghee instead of coconut oil. ●

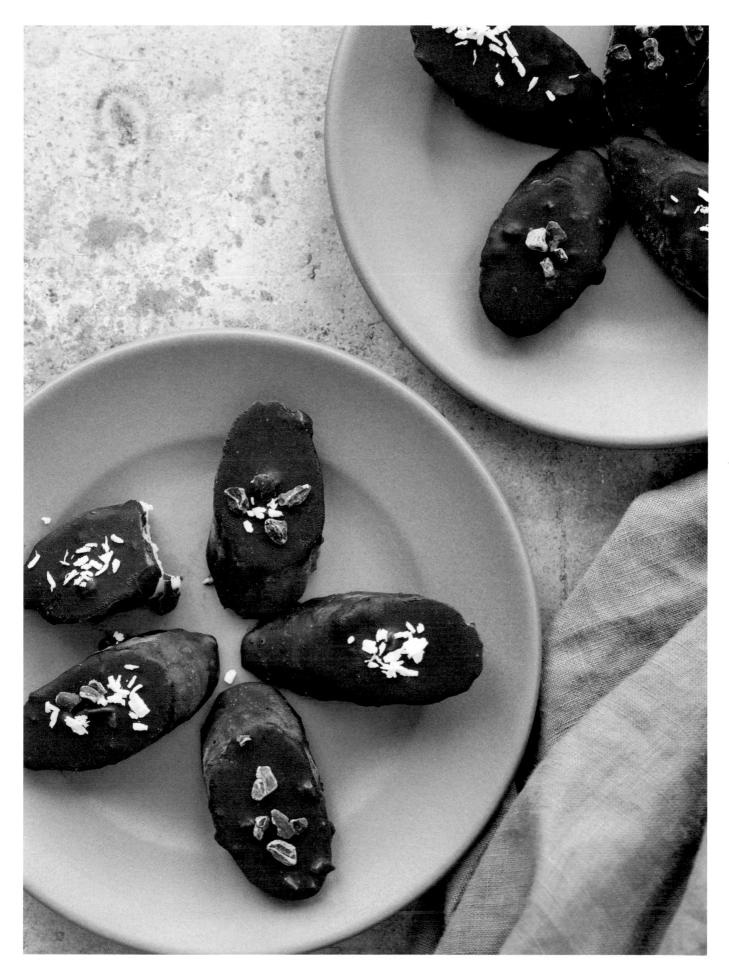

21DSD Fudge Pops

PREP TIME **5 MINUTES, PLUS OVERNIGHT TO FREEZE** • COOK TIME — •
MAKES **4 TWIN-SIZED POPS (1 PER SERVING)**

NUTS
EGGS
NIGHTSHADES
FODMAPS

1 cup almond milk, store-bought or homemade (page 242)

1 medium green-tipped banana

3 tablespoons unsweetened carob powder or cocoa powder

2 tablespoons almond butter

Pinch of ground cinnamon

Cacao nibs, for garnish (optional)

SPECIAL EQUIPMENT

Ice pop molds

Purée all the ingredients in a blender until smooth.

If using cacao nibs, sprinkle a few into the bottom of each pop mold.

Pour the blended mixture evenly into the molds, insert your popsicle sticks, and freeze overnight.

To remove the pops, run the molds under warm water until the sides release.

21DSD FRUIT SERVING
Each serving includes about a quarter of a banana. Factor this into your total intake of allowed fruit for the day. ●

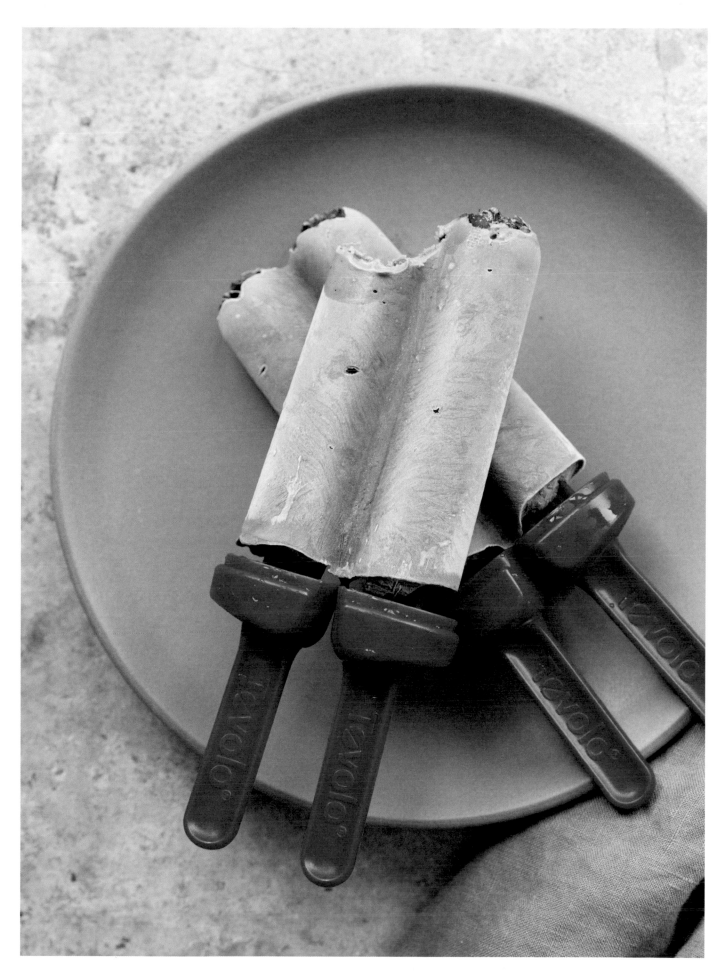

Lemon Vanilla Meltaways

PREP TIME **10 MINUTES, PLUS 20 MINUTES TO CHILL** • COOK TIME —
• MAKES **12 PIECES (3 PER SERVING)**

NUTS
EGGS
NIGHTSHADES
FODMAPS

1/2 cup coconut
   butter, softened
1/2 cup coconut
   oil, softened
Seeds scraped from 1/2
   vanilla bean pod
Grated zest and
   juice of 1 lemon

SPECIAL EQUIPMENT
1 (12-cavity) mini-muffin tin
12 parchment paper mini
   baking cups

Line a 12-cavity mini-muffin tin with mini parchment paper baking cups.

In a mixing bowl (preferably one with a spout), whisk together the coconut butter, coconut oil, vanilla bean seeds, lemon zest, and lemon juice until well combined.

Pour the mixture into the prepared muffin tin and chill for 20 to 30 minutes, until completely solid.

KITCHEN TIP
Parchment paper baking cups are critical to keep the meltaways from sticking to the pan. They're easy to find at most grocery stores, or they can easily be ordered online on a site like Amazon. ●

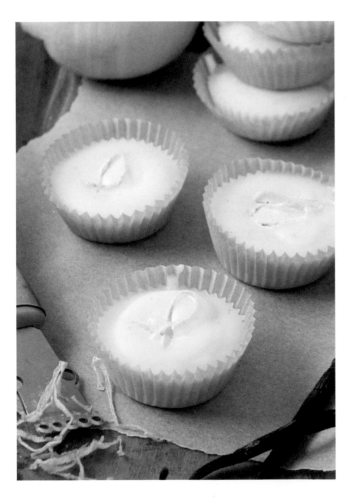

Granny Smith Apple Crumble

PREP TIME **15 MINUTES** • COOK TIME **45 TO 50 MINUTES** • MAKES **4 SERVINGS**

FOR THE FILLING

4 green apples, peeled and thinly sliced

Juice of 1/2 lemon

1 teaspoon ground cinnamon

FOR THE TOPPING

1 1/4 cups almond meal, store-bought or homemade (page 242), or other nut meal

1/4 cup unsalted butter or coconut oil, softened

1 teaspoon ground cinnamon

Pinch of sea salt

1 tablespoon unsalted butter or coconut oil, melted, for the pan

NUTS

EGGS

NIGHTSHADES

FODMAPS

Preheat the oven to 350°F.

Make the filling: In a large mixing bowl, toss the apples with the lemon juice and cinnamon.

Make the topping: In a separate large mixing bowl, mix together the almond meal, 1/4 cup butter, cinnamon, and salt until completely incorporated.

Brush the bottom and sides of a 9 by 9-inch baking dish with the melted butter. Place the apples in the baking dish and cover evenly with the topping. Cover the dish with foil.

Bake for 20 minutes, then remove the foil cover and bake for an additional 25 to 30 minutes, until the apples are soft and the topping begins to brown on the edges.

CHEF NOTE

If you're like me, you'll find yourself returning to this recipe even after you've completed the 21DSD. It's the perfect super-simple after-dinner treat that's not too sweet. ●

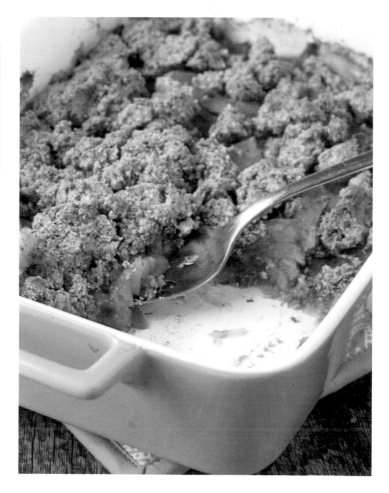

SAUCES
DRESSINGS
& BASICS

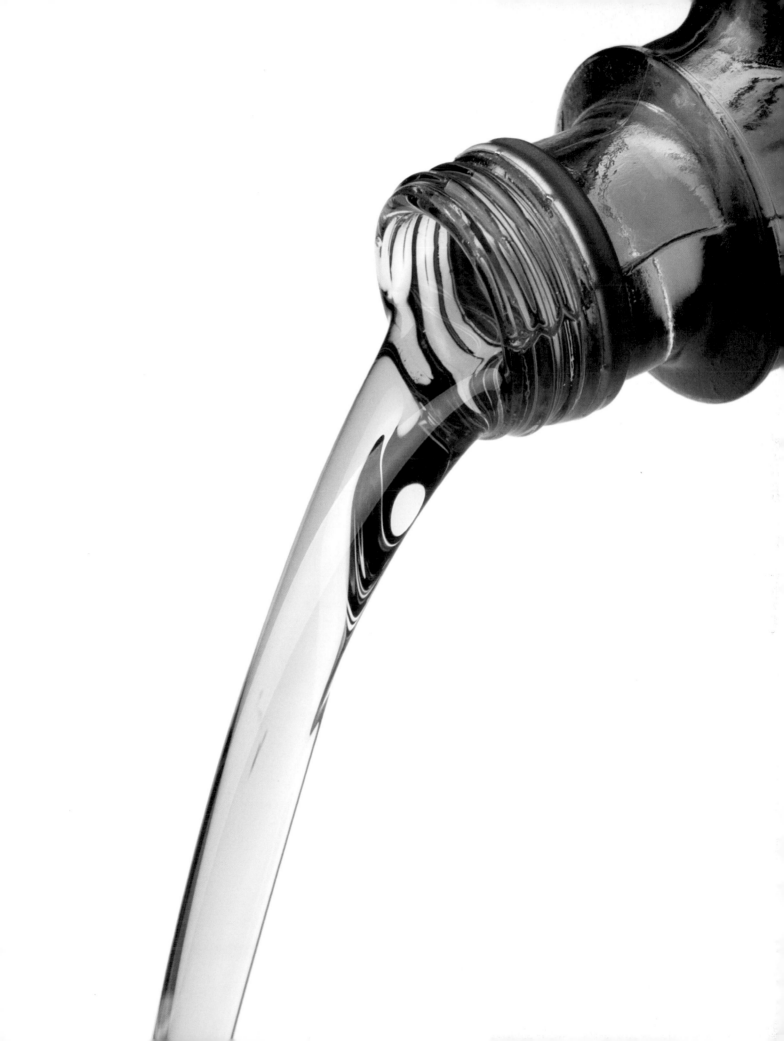

Perfectly Grilled Chicken Breast

PREP TIME **10 MINUTES, PLUS 5 MINUTES TO MARINATE**
• COOK TIME **10 MINUTES** • MAKES **4 SERVINGS**

NUTS
EGGS
NIGHTSHADES
FODMAPS

1 pound boneless, skinless chicken breast

Juice of 1 lemon, or 2 tablespoons balsamic vinegar

1 teaspoon dried oregano, rosemary, or other herb

1/2 teaspoon sea salt

1/2 teaspoon ground black pepper

2 tablespoons coconut oil or ghee

2 tablespoons extra-virgin olive oil

Preheat a grill pan or grill to medium heat.

Place a chicken breast on a cutting board with the thickest side facing you. Set your non-cutting hand on top and, while pressing down slightly on the chicken with your palm (keeping your fingers out straight), begin cutting down the length of the side of the breast, keeping your knife parallel to the cutting board. Carefully slide the knife through the center of the breast so that the thickness is cut in half.

Continue to slice almost completely through the chicken breast, leaving it connected in the center so that it flattens out to a butterfly or heart shape. The chicken should now be 1/4- to 1/2-inch thick, at most. Repeat with the remaining chicken breasts.

In a large bowl, combine the lemon juice with the oregano, salt, and pepper. Add the chicken and turn to evenly coat. Marinate for at least 5 minutes, but not more than an hour.

Brush the hot grill or grill pan with the coconut oil, then cook the chicken for 4 to 5 minutes per side, depending on the thickness of the chicken. When the chicken has turned white around the sides and toward the middle, it's time to flip it.

Remove the chicken from the heat and brush it liberally with the olive oil. Allow to rest for at least 5 minutes before slicing.

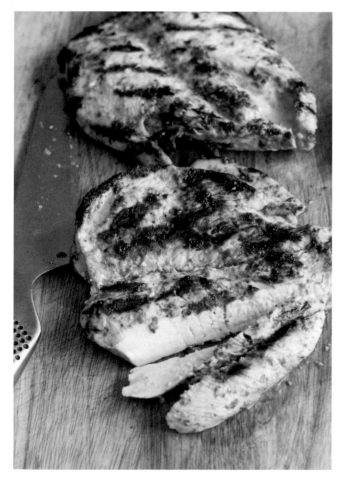

Caramelized Onions

PREP TIME **10 MINUTES** • COOK TIME **45 MINUTES** • MAKES **ABOUT 1 CUP**

2 tablespoons cooking fat

4 small onions (yellow, red, or a combination), thinly sliced

1/2 teaspoon sea salt

1/2 teaspoon dried rosemary or thyme (optional)

NUTS

EGGS

NIGHTSHADES

FODMAPS

In a large sauté pan or skillet over medium heat, melt the cooking fat, then place the onions in the pan. Cook the onions for 8 to 10 minutes, until they begin to become translucent, then add the salt and dried herbs, if using.

Reduce the heat to medium-low and slowly cook the onions, stirring occasionally, allowing them to brown just slightly before stirring each time. If you find that the onions are browning too quickly or are sticking too much, reduce the heat slightly, add 1 to 2 tablespoons of warm water at a time to the pan, and stir it into the onions to keep them cooking evenly. Over the cooking time, the onions will become more and more browned and softened, and eventually they will look as they do in the photo. They will be rich-tasting and richly colored at the end of cooking, around 45 minutes. This process requires low, slow heat; faster, hotter heat will not yield the same results.

CHANGE IT UP
Add 1 to 2 tablespoons of balsamic vinegar to the onions for the last 10 minutes of cooking for a more robust flavor.

CHEF NOTE
Enjoy these onions as a topping for burgers, sausages, or grass-fed hot dogs, or mixed into meatloaf or omelets. ●

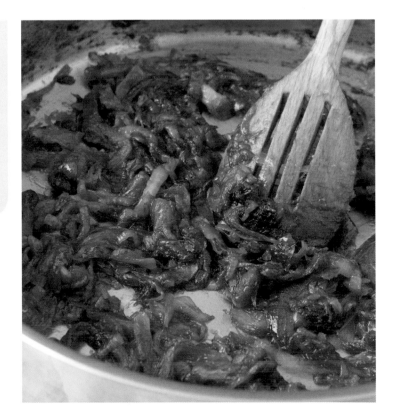

21DSD Ketchup

PREP TIME **10 MINUTES** • COOK TIME **4 HOURS IN A SLOW COOKER** • MAKES **2 CUPS**

NUTS

EGGS

NIGHTSHADES

FODMAPS

1 small onion, diced

2 green apples, peeled and diced

2 cloves garlic, minced

1/4 cup water

2 tablespoons apple cider vinegar

1/2 teaspoon sea salt

1/4 teaspoon allspice

1/4 teaspoon ground cinnamon

1/4 teaspoon ginger powder

2 pinches of ground cloves

6 ounces tomato paste

Place all the ingredients in a slow cooker and stir to combine. Set the slow cooker to low and cook for 4 hours.

Allow the mixture to cool slightly, then pour into a food processor or high-speed blender and blend until smooth.

Once blended, place the ketchup in glass jars and allow it to come to room temperature before refrigerating.

The ketchup should last for several weeks or more in the refrigerator. If you notice a change in color or smell or see any mold growth, toss it and make a new batch.

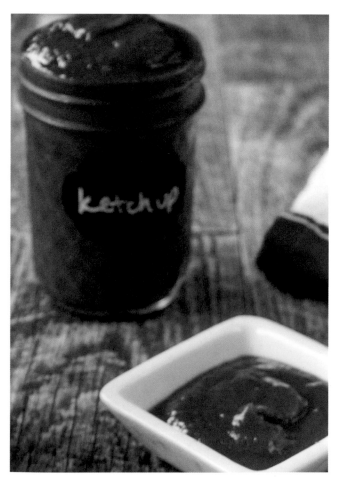

KITCHEN TIP
When blending or processing warm foods, do not overfill the container, as the heat will cause the contents to expand and they may splatter out. ●

21DSD BBQ Sauce

PREP TIME **10 MINUTES, PLUS ABOUT 1 HOUR FOR THE CARAMELIZED ONIONS**
• COOK TIME — • MAKES **2 CUPS**

2 cups 21DSD Ketchup (page 232)

1/2 cup Caramelized Onions (page 231)

1/4 cup apple cider vinegar

1 teaspoon mustard powder

1/2 to 1 teaspoon chipotle powder, or less for less heat (see Note)

1/2 teaspoon paprika

1/2 teaspoon sea salt

1/4 to 1/2 cup water (optional)

Combine all the ingredients except the water in a blender and blend on high for 2 to 3 minutes, until well combined.

If you prefer a thinner consistency, add the water and blend for 1 more minute. Taste and add more chipotle powder if desired.

Store in a glass jar in the refrigerator for up to 5 days.

NUTS

EGGS

NIGHTSHADES

FODMAPS

NOTE
The newer your chipotle powder is, the hotter it will be! Pepper spices lose their punch as they age, so start with the smaller amount if your batch is new. ●

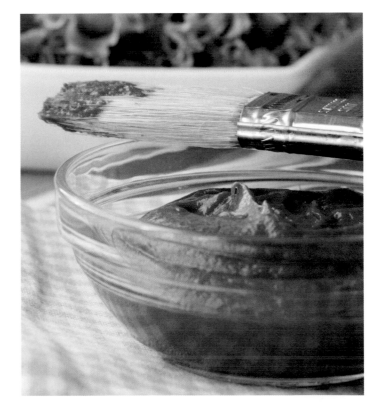

Peanut Sauce

PREP TIME **5 MINUTES** • COOK TIME **—** • MAKES **1 1/4 CUPS**

NUTS
EGGS
NIGHTSHADES
FODMAPS

1/2 cup peanut butter or other nut or seed butter

1/2 cup coconut aminos

1/4 cup rice vinegar

2 to 3 dashes of fish sauce

1/2 teaspoon sesame seeds

1/4 teaspoon sea salt

1/4 teaspoon ground black pepper

1/4 teaspoon red pepper flakes (optional)

Combine all the ingredients in a small mixing bowl and whisk together vigorously.

Store in a glass jar in the refrigerator for up to 2 weeks.

VARIATION: PEANUT DRESSING
Add the juice of 1 to 2 limes or some water to thin the sauce further to make it into a salad dressing.

NUT-FREE?
Use tahini (ground sesame seeds) instead of peanut butter.

NIGHTSHADE-FREE?
Omit the red pepper flakes.

CHANGE IT UP
If you are allergic to seafood, omit the fish sauce. ●

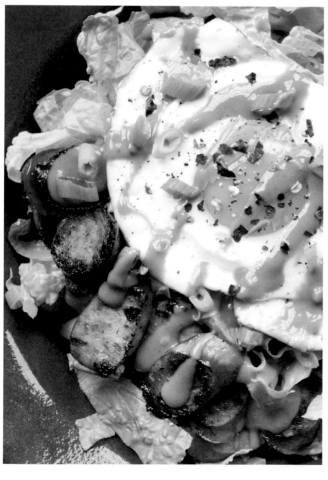

Cashew "Cheese" Sauce

PREP TIME **5 MINUTES, PLUS AT LEAST 1 HOUR TO SOAK THE CASHEWS**
• COOK TIME — • MAKES **1 1/2 TO 2 CUPS (ABOUT 8 SERVINGS)**

1 cup raw cashews

1 cup water

1 cup nutritional yeast (see page 127)

1/4 cup peeled and cooked sweet potato

1 teaspoon sea salt

1 teaspoon garlic powder

1 teaspoon onion powder

1/2 teaspoon ground black pepper

1/2 teaspoon paprika

Place the cashews in a medium-sized container, cover completely with warm water, and soak for 1 to 4 hours unrefrigerated or up to overnight refrigerated.

Drain the cashews, then add to a blender with the other ingredients. Blend until smooth. If the sauce is too thick, add more water, 2 tablespoons at a time, until the desired consistency is reached.

Store in an airtight container in the fridge for up to 5 days. Freeze leftovers a in a freezer-safe bag until needed. Blend again if necessary after defrosting.

NUTS

EGGS

NIGHTSHADES

FODMAPS

NIGHTSHADE-FREE?
Omit the paprika.

KITCHEN TIP
If you need to soak the cashews overnight but won't be able to prepare the recipe until later the next day, drain them in the morning and store them in the refrigerator until you are ready to make the sauce. When you make the sauce, be sure to use warm water for blending. ●

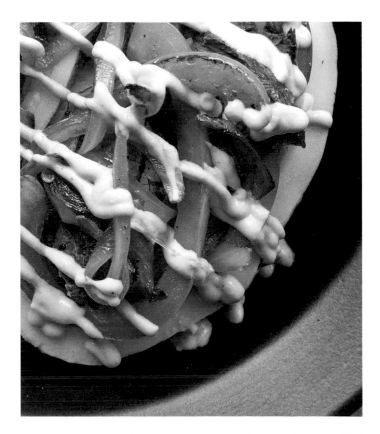

Pesto Sauce

PREP TIME **10 MINUTES** • COOK TIME **—** • MAKES **1 1/2 CUPS**

NUTS
EGGS
NIGHTSHADES
FODMAPS

2 cups tightly packed fresh
  basil leaves

2 large cloves garlic, peeled

1/4 cup pine nuts, or
  1/2 cup walnut halves

1/4 cup shredded
  hard cheese, such as
  Parmigiano-Reggiano or
  Pecorino Romano (Levels
  1 & 2 only; see Note)

1/4 teaspoon sea salt

1/4 teaspoon ground black
  pepper

1/2 cup extra-virgin olive oil

Combine the basil, garlic, nuts, cheese, salt, and
pepper in a food processor and blend until smooth.
Add the olive oil and continue to blend until
smooth. Taste and add more salt and pepper if
needed.

Store in an airtight container in the fridge for up to
2 weeks.

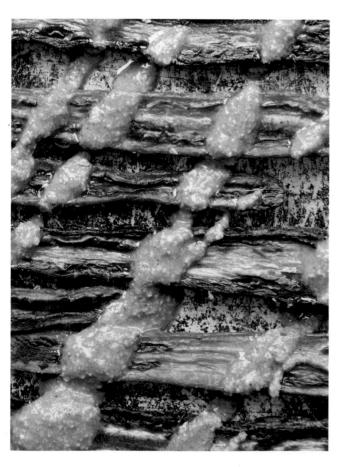

NOTE
If you're on Level 3, use 1/4 cup nutritional
yeast (see page 127) instead of cheese. ●

Simple Marinara

PREP TIME **10 MINUTES** • COOK TIME **30 MINUTES** • MAKES **ABOUT 3 CUPS**

2 tablespoons cooking fat

1/2 cup diced yellow onion

Sea salt and ground black pepper

2 or 3 cloves garlic, grated or minced

1 (28-ounce) can diced tomatoes

1 tablespoon chopped fresh basil leaves

2 tablespoons extra-virgin olive oil, to finish

In a saucepan, melt the cooking fat over medium heat. Add the onion and cook until it is translucent, approximately 5 minutes. Season with salt and pepper.

Add the garlic and cook for an additional 30 seconds. Add the tomatoes, season with additional salt and pepper, and stir to combine. Reduce the heat to low and simmer for 15 to 20 minutes.

Add the basil and simmer for an additional 5 minutes.

Drizzle with the olive oil before serving. Store in an airtight container in the refrigerator for up to 5 days.

NUTS

EGGS

NIGHTSHADES

FODMAPS

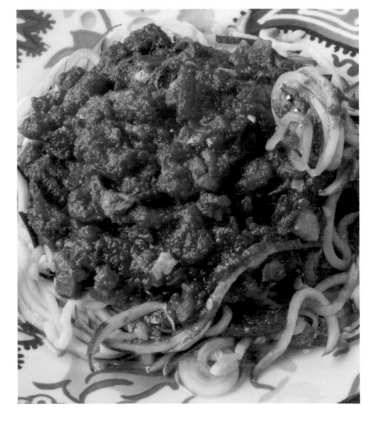

Balsamic Vinaigrette Dressing

PREP TIME **5 MINUTES** • COOK TIME **—** • MAKES **1 CUP (ABOUT 8 SERVINGS)**

NUTS
EGGS
NIGHTSHADES
FODMAPS

- 2/3 cup extra-virgin olive oil
- 1/3 cup balsamic vinegar
- 1 teaspoon gluten-free Dijon mustard
- 1/2 teaspoon minced shallot or garlic
- 1/2 teaspoon dried oregano or basil (optional)
- 1/4 teaspoon sea salt
- 1/4 teaspoon ground black pepper

Combine all the ingredients in a glass jar with a lid and shake well to combine.

Label and store in the refrigerator for up to a month.

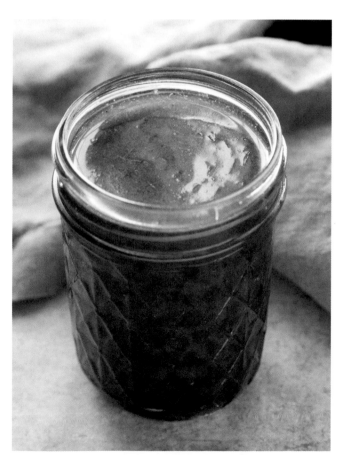

Lemon-Herb Dressing

PREP TIME **5 MINUTES** • COOK TIME **—** • MAKES **1 CUP (ABOUT 8 SERVINGS)**

2/3 cup extra-virgin olive oil

1/3 cup fresh lemon juice

1 teaspoon gluten-free Dijon mustard

1/2 teaspoon minced shallot

1/2 teaspoon minced fresh cilantro or basil (optional)

1/4 teaspoon sea salt

1/4 teaspoon ground black pepper

Combine all the ingredients in a glass jar with a lid and shake well to combine.

Label and store in the refrigerator for up to a month.

NUTS

EGGS

NIGHTSHADES

FODMAPS

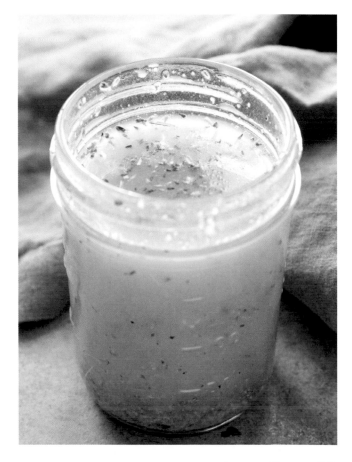

Ranch Dressing

PREP TIME **5 MINUTES** • COOK TIME — • MAKES **3/4 CUP**

NUTS

EGGS

NIGHTSHADES

FODMAPS

3/4 cup coconut cream (see page 126)

3 tablespoons fresh lemon juice (1 medium lemon)

3 tablespoons Ranch Spice Blend (page 249)

2 tablespoons extra-virgin olive oil

1 heaping tablespoon chopped fresh chives (optional)

1/2 teaspoon apple cider vinegar

1/2 teaspoon minced or grated garlic (about 1 clove)

1/2 teaspoon crushed red pepper (optional)

In a small mixing bowl, whisk together all the ingredients.

If you prefer a thicker dressing, chill it in the refrigerator before serving.

Store in an airtight container in the fridge for up to a week.

KITCHEN TIPS

If the dressing is too firm after refrigerating, simply whisk in 1 tablespoon of warm water. You can use lemon juice instead if you like it more tart.

When adding raw garlic to a dressing, sauce, or dip that remains uncooked, more is not always better! The potency of raw garlic will intensify in recipes as it sits, so don't let this recipe be one where you read "1 clove" and translate it to "4 cloves" as garlic lovers often do when cooking!

NIGHTSHADE-FREE?

Omit the red pepper flakes. ●

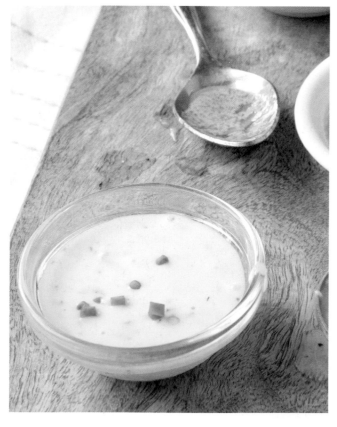

Basic Cilantro Cauli-Rice

PREP TIME **15 MINUTES** • COOK TIME **5 OR 10 MINUTES** • MAKES **4 SERVINGS**

1 head cauliflower, cut into florets

1/4 cup minced red onion (optional)

1/4 cup minced yellow bell pepper (optional)

1 or 2 tablespoons coconut oil or bacon fat

Sea salt and ground black pepper

1/4 cup finely chopped fresh cilantro leaves

Cilantro sprig, for garnish (optional)

Grate the cauliflower using a box grater or food processor.

If using red onion and yellow bell pepper, sauté them in 1 tablespoon of coconut oil in a small skillet over medium heat for about 5 minutes, or until they become soft and have golden-brown edges.

In a large skillet over medium heat, melt 1 tablespoon of coconut oil. Add the grated cauliflower to the skillet and season with salt and pepper. Sauté for about 5 minutes, or until the cauliflower begins to become translucent, stirring gently to ensure that it cooks through. Stir in the cooked onion and bell pepper, if using.

Transfer the cooked cauliflower to a serving bowl and toss with the chopped cilantro before serving. Garnish with a sprig of cilantro if desired.

NUTS

EGGS

NIGHTSHADES

FODMAPS

NIGHTSHADE-FREE?
Omit the bell pepper. ●

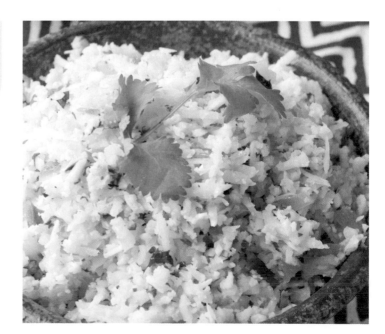

Almond Milk & Meal

PREP TIME 10 MINUTES, PLUS 8 HOURS TO SOAK THE ALMONDS
• COOK TIME — • MAKES **2 CUPS**

NUTS
EGGS
NIGHTSHADES
FODMAPS

2 cups raw almonds
7 cups water, divided

OPTIONAL FLAVORINGS
1/2 to 1 teaspoon
  pure vanilla extract
  (recommended)
1/2 teaspoon ground
  cinnamon
1/2 teaspoon unsweetened
  cocoa powder

SPECIAL EQUIPMENT
Nut milk bag or
  cheesecloth

To make almond milk: Place the almonds and 4 cups of the water in a glass or other nonporous container and soak, covered, in a dark place for 8 hours or overnight.

Drain and rinse the almonds in clean water.

Place the rinsed almonds in a blender with the remaining 3 cups of water and blend on high for 2 minutes. Strain the liquid through a nut milk bag or layered cheesecloth over a bowl to catch the milk. Reserve the strained meal.

If using optional flavorings, rinse out the blender, place the milk back in with the flavorings, and pulse to combine.

Store the almond milk in the refrigerator for up to 5 days.

To make almond meal: Preheat the oven to 170°F to 200°F. Dehydrate the strained meal on a rimmed baking sheet for 3 to 4 hours, until completely dry. Pulse in a food processor to smooth out the clumps. Store in the refrigerator for up to 3 weeks.

KITCHEN TIP
This recipe works best in a powerful high-speed blender like a Blendtec or Vitamix. ●

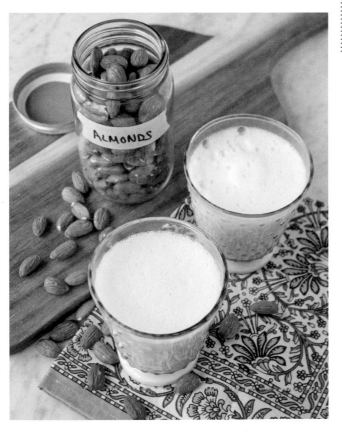

Coconut Milk & Flour

PREP TIME **10 MINUTES, PLUS 30 MINUTES TO SOAK THE COCONUT FLAKES** •
COOK TIME — • MAKES **4 CUPS**

2 cups unsweetened
  coconut flakes

4 cups water, divided

1 teaspoon pure vanilla
  extract

In a medium-sized bowl, combine the coconut flakes and 2 cups of warm (not hot) water. Let sit for at least 30 minutes to soften the coconut flakes.

Put the coconut flakes and soaking water in a blender and add 2 more cups of water. Blend on high for about 1 minute, or until the coconut is fully blended into the water.

If you have a nut milk bag, pour the contents of the blender into the bag and squeeze all the milk into a large bowl. Transfer the milk to a resealable glass container, add the vanilla, and stir to combine.

If you don't have a nut milk bag, use a fine-mesh strainer to strain the milk, pushing the solids against the sides to get as much liquid out as possible.

Reserve the strained solids. Store the milk in an airtight glass container in the refrigerator for up to 5 days.

To make coconut flour: Preheat the oven to 200°F. Spread out the coconut solids in an even layer on a rimmed baking sheet, breaking up the larger pieces. Turn off the oven and place the baking sheet in the oven overnight. Place the dehydrated coconut in a food processor and process for approximately 1 to 2 minutes, until finely ground. Store in the refrigerator for up to 3 weeks.

NUTS

EGGS

NIGHTSHADES

FODMAPS

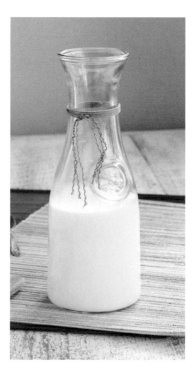

KITCHEN TIPS

This recipe works best in a powerful high-speed blender like a Blendtec or Vitamix.

If you're not making coconut flour, you can use the reserved solids from making coconut milk to add healthy fats and nutrients to smoothies. ●

Bone Broth

PREP TIME **5 MINUTES** • COOK TIME **AT LEAST 8 HOURS IN A SLOW COOKER** •
MAKES **ABOUT 2 1/2 QUARTS**

NUTS

EGGS

NIGHTSHADES

FODMAPS

4 quarts filtered water

1 1/2 to 2 pounds bones (beef knuckle bones, marrow bones, meaty bones, chicken or turkey necks, chicken or turkey bones, or any bones you have on hand)

2 tablespoons apple cider vinegar

2 teaspoons sea salt

Cloves from 1 head garlic, peeled and smashed (optional)

Place all the ingredients in a 6-quart slow cooker. Turn the heat to high and bring the water to a boil. Then reduce the heat to low. Allow the broth to cook for a minimum of 8 hours and up to 24 hours. The longer it cooks, the better.

Turn off the slow cooker and allow the broth to cool to room temperature. Strain the broth through a fine-mesh strainer or a colander lined with cheesecloth. Store in glass jars in the refrigerator for up to a week or in the freezer for up to several months.

Before using the broth, chip away at the top and discard any fat that has solidified. You can drink the broth or use it as a base for soups, stews, or any recipe that calls for stock or broth.

FODMAP-FREE?
Omit the garlic. ●

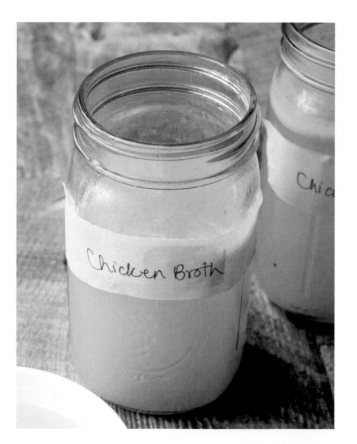

Vegetable Broth

PREP TIME **15 MINUTES** • COOK TIME **AT LEAST 4 HOURS IN A SLOW COOKER** • MAKES **ABOUT 2 1/2 QUARTS**

1 large onion, chopped

4 large carrots, chopped

4 large celery stalks, chopped

8 cloves garlic, peeled and smashed

2 bay leaves

2 teaspoons sea salt

4 quarts filtered water

6 to 8 sprigs fresh parsley and/or thyme (optional)

Place all the ingredients in a 6-quart slow cooker. Turn the heat to high and bring the water to a boil. Then reduce the heat to low and cook the broth for a minimum of 4 hours and a maximum of 8 hours. The longer it cooks, the more flavorful it will become.

Turn off the slow cooker and allow the broth to cool to room temperature. Strain the broth through a fine-mesh strainer or a colander lined with cheesecloth and discard the solids. Place in glass jars and store in the refrigerator for up to a week or in the freezer for up to several months.

NUTS

EGGS

NIGHTSHADES

FODMAPS

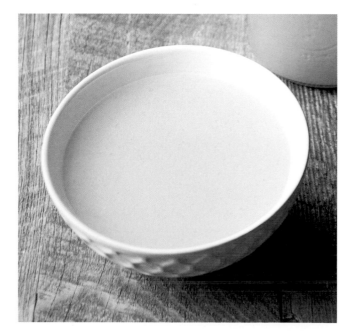

Healthy Homemade Mayonnaise

PREP TIME **15 MINUTES** • COOK TIME — • MAKES **3/4 CUP**

NUTS
EGGS
NIGHTSHADES
FODMAPS

2 egg yolks

1 tablespoon fresh lemon juice

1 teaspoon gluten-free Dijon mustard

1/2 cup macadamia nut oil or other oil

1/4 cup extra-virgin olive oil

In a medium-sized mixing bowl, whisk together the egg yolks, lemon juice, and mustard until blended and bright yellow, about 30 seconds.

Add 1/4 cup of the macadamia nut oil to the yolk mixture a few drops at a time, whisking constantly. Gradually add the remaining 1/4 cup macadamia nut oil and the olive oil in a slow, thin stream, whisking constantly, until the mayonnaise is thick and lighter in color.

Store in the refrigerator for up to a week.

KITCHEN TIP
You can also make this recipe using a handheld immersion blender or a small blender. If using a regular-sized blender, double the recipe to make blending easier. Use the opening at the top of your blender to slowly drizzle in the oil. ●

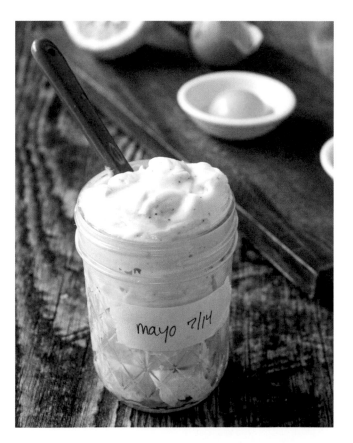

Clarified Butter & Ghee

PREP TIME **5 MINUTES** · COOK TIME **25 TO 30 MINUTES (CLARIFIED BUTTER), 35 TO 45 MINUTES (GHEE)** · MAKES **25 TO 30 FLUID OUNCES**

2 pounds unsalted butter from pastured cows (brands I like include Kerrygold, SMJÖR, Organic Pastures, and Organic Valley Pasture Butter)

SPECIAL EQUIPMENT
Cheesecloth

To make clarified butter: Slowly melt the butter in a medium-sized heavy-bottomed saucepan over low heat. As the butter comes to a simmer, the milk solids will float to the top and become foamy while the separated oil will become very clear. Skim off the milk solids and remove the clarified butter from the heat. Pour it through cheesecloth to strain out any remaining milk solids, and store the strained liquid in a glass jar.

To make ghee: Follow the instructions for making clarified butter, but allow the milk solids to continue to cook slowly until they become browned and begin to sink to the bottom of the pan. When there are no longer any solids waiting to brown and sink to the bottom, the ghee is finished. Pour it through cheesecloth to strain out the browned milk solids, and store the strained liquid in a glass jar.

With all the milk solids removed, clarified butter and ghee are stable oils that will keep indefinitely.

NUTS

EGGS

NIGHTSHADES

FODMAPS

KEEP IT COOL, OR DON'T
When all the milk solids are removed, clarified butter and ghee are shelf stable and will last indefinitely in the pantry. However, if some milk solids remain and the temperature in your home becomes very warm, they may go off. To prevent this, store them in the refrigerator— just be aware that they'll become solid. ●

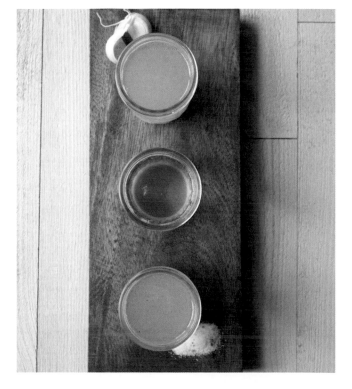

Spice Blends

For each blend, combine all of the ingredients in a small bowl. Store in a small airtight container in a cool, dark place for up to a year. Use these blends as they appear in recipes throughout the book—or anytime! To order my premade spice blends online, visit 21DSD.com/spices.

BBQ SPICE BLEND
Makes about 1/2 cup

3 tablespoons paprika
1 1/2 tablespoons chili powder
1 1/2 tablespoons granulated garlic
1 1/2 tablespoons granulated onion
1 1/2 teaspoons sea salt
1 1/2 teaspoons ground black pepper
1/2 teaspoon ground cinnamon

SMOKY SPICE BLEND
Makes 1/2 cup

2 tablespoons smoked paprika
2 tablespoons granulated onion
1 tablespoon chipotle powder
1 tablespoon sea salt
1 tablespoon sweet paprika
1 1/2 teaspoons ground cinnamon
1 1/2 teaspoons ground black pepper

GREEK SPICE BLEND
Makes about 1/2 cup

3 tablespoons dried oregano leaves
2 1/2 tablespoons granulated garlic
2 tablespoons dried lemon peel
1 1/2 teaspoons sea salt
1 teaspoon ground black pepper

TACO & FAJITA SPICE BLEND
Makes 1/2 cup

2 tablespoons chili powder
1 1/2 tablespoons granulated garlic
1 1/2 tablespoons granulated onion
1 tablespoon ground coriander
2 teaspoons ground cumin
2 teaspoons smoked paprika
1 teaspoon sea salt
1 teaspoon ground black pepper

ITALIAN SPICE BLEND
Makes about 1/2 cup

3 tablespoons dried parsley
1 1/2 tablespoons granulated garlic
1 tablespoon granulated onion
1 tablespoon fennel seeds, roughly chopped
1 tablespoon dried ground sage
1 teaspoon ground black pepper or 1/4 teaspoon ground white pepper
1 teaspoon sea salt

NOTE
Use 2 tablespoons of Italian Spice Blend per pound of meat to make sausage. ●

EVERYTHING BAGEL SPICE BLEND
Makes 1 cup

5 tablespoons dried garlic flakes
3 1/3 tablespoons poppy seeds
3 1/3 tablespoons dried onion flakes
3 tablespoons sesame seeds
1 tablespoon coarse sea salt

RANCH SPICE BLEND
Makes about 1 cup

5 1/2 tablespoons dried garlic flakes
2 1/2 tablespoons dill weed
2 1/2 tablespoons dried chives
2 1/2 tablespoons dried parsley
1 tablespoon sea salt
2 1/2 teaspoons ground mustard
2 1/2 teaspoons dried lemon peel
1 1/2 teaspoons celery powder

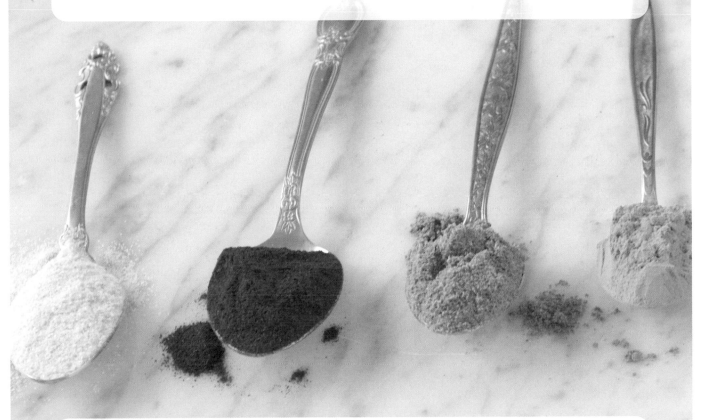

SUPER GARLIC SPICE BLEND
Makes 1 cup

9 tablespoons dried garlic flakes
4 tablespoons dried chives
2 tablespoons granulated garlic
1 1/2 tablespoons sea salt

TRIFECTA SPICE BLEND
Makes about 1 cup

10 tablespoons granulated garlic
5 1/3 tablespoons sea salt
2 tablespoons ground black pepper

RESOURCES

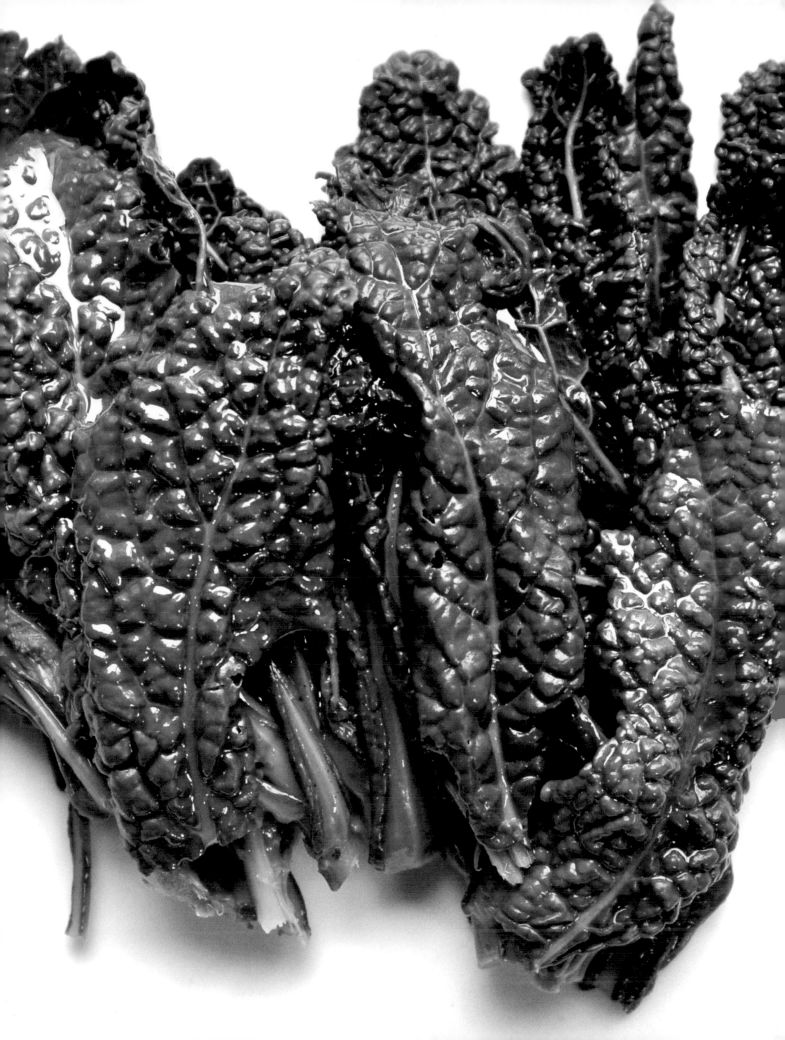

RECIPE ALLERGEN INDEX

Recipe	pg	NUT-FREE	EGG-FREE	NIGHTSHADES-FREE	FODMAP-FREE
Breakfast Salad	130				●
Apple Cinnamon Muffins	132			●	
Mushroom, Pesto & Goat Cheese Frittata	134			●	
Broccoli, Ham & Cheese Frittata	136	●		●	M
Sausage, Spinach & Peppers Frittata	138	●			
Bacon, Brussels, Asparagus & Goat Cheese Frittata	140	●		●	M
Banana Nut Smoothie	142		●	●	
Apple Pie Smoothie	144	M	●	●	
Pumpkin Spice Smoothie	145		●	●	
Banana Vanilla Bean N'Oatmeal	146	●	M	●	
Grain-Free Banola	147			●	
Bacon & Root Veggie Hash	148	●	●	●	M
Pumpkin Pancakes with Vanilla Bean Coconut Butter	149	●		●	
B3 Bowl	152	●	●		
BBQ Burgers with Spicy Slaw	154	●	●		●
BBQ Chicken Salad	156		●		
BBQ Pulled Pork Tacos with Spicy Slaw	158	●	●	M	
Slow Cooker BBQ Pulled Pork	158	●	●	M	
BBQ Pulled Pork Buddha Bowl	160	●	●		
Buffalo Cauliflower & Chicken Wings	162	●	●		
Chicken Fajita Salad	164	●	●		
Ranch Chicken & Bacon Stuffed Potatoes	166	●	●	●	
Cheesesteak Stuffed Potatoes	168		●		
Diane's Simple Roast Chicken	170	●	●	●	M
Smoky Chicken Salad Lettuce Boats	172	●	M		
Creamy Mustard Chicken with Zoodles	174	●	●	●	
Tangy Chicken Salad	176	●	●	M	
Deli Tuna Sliders	178	●	M	M	
Mediterranean Meatball Bowl	180	●	●	M	
Grilled Pork Fall Salad	182	M	●		M
Super Garlic Meatballs with Fried Rice	184	●	●	M	
Sausage & Spinach "Polenta" Bowl	186	●	●		
Super Garlic Salmon & Vegetables	188	●	●	●	
Simple Fried Rice	192	●	●		
Crispy Brussels Sprouts	194	●	●	●	
Garlic Butter Sautéed Mushrooms	196	●	●	●	
Pesto Roasted Carrots	198		●	●	
Crispy Broccoli	200	●	●	M	
Roasted Butternut Squash	202	●	●	●	
Roasted Garlic Cauliflower Polenta	204	●	●	●	
Ranch Roasted Potatoes	206	●	●	M	
Roasted Eggplant Steaks with Tahini Sauce	208	M	●		M
Simple Deviled Eggs	210	●		M	
Smoky Toasted Nut Mix	212		●		
Cinilla Nut Mix	214			●	

M can be modified to be free of this allergen

Recipe	pg	NUT-FREE	EGG-FREE	NIGHTSHADES-FREE	FODMAP-FREE
Spicy Thai Nut Mix	214		●	●	
Simple Beef Jerky	215	●	●	●	
Two-Bite Chocolate Cream Pies	218		●	●	
21DSD Cinnamon Banana Bread	220			●	
21DSD Frozen Coco-Monkey Bites	222	M	●	●	M
21DSD Fudge Pops	224		●	●	
Lemon Vanilla Meltaways	226	●	●	●	
Granny Smith Apple Crumble	227		●	●	
Perfectly Grilled Chicken Breast	230	●	●	●	●
Caramelized Onions	231	●	●	●	
21DSD Ketchup	232	●	●		
21DSD BBQ Sauce	233	●	●		
Peanut Sauce	234	M	●	M	●
Cashew "Cheese" Sauce	235		●	M	
Pesto Sauce	236		●	●	
Simple Marinara	237	●	●		
Balsamic Vinaigrette Dressing	238	●	●	●	
Lemon-Herb Dressing	239	●	●	●	
Ranch Dressing	240	●	●	M	
Basic Cilantro Cauli-Rice	241	●	●	M	
Almond Milk & Meal	242		●	●	●
Coconut Milk & Flour	243	●	●	●	
Bone Broth	244	●	●	●	M
Vegetable Broth	245	●	●	●	M
Healthy Homemade Mayonnaise	246	●		●	●
Clarified Butter & Ghee	247	●	●	●	●

M can be modified to be free of this allergen

RECIPE INDEX

BREAKFAST

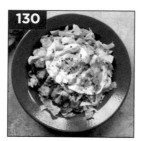
130
Breakfast Salad

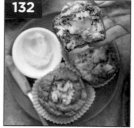
132
Apple Cinnamon Muffins

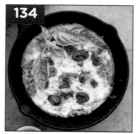
134
Mushroom, Pesto & Goat Cheese Frittata

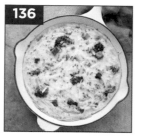
136
Broccoli, Ham & Cheese Frittata

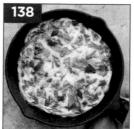
138
Sausage, Spinach & Peppers Frittata

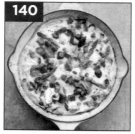
140
Bacon, Brussels, Asparagus & Goat Cheese Frittata

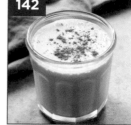
142
Banana Nut Smoothie

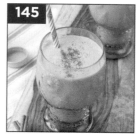
144
Apple Pie Smoothie

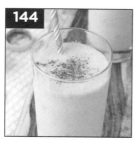
145
Pumpkin Spice Smoothie

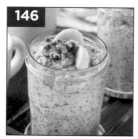
146
Banana Vanilla Bean N'Oatmeal

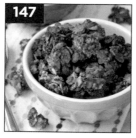
147
Grain-Free Banola

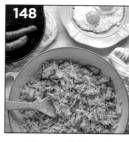
148
Bacon & Root Veggie Hash

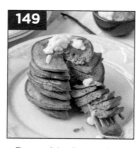
149
Pumpkin Pancakes with Vanilla Bean Coconut Butter

MAIN DISHES

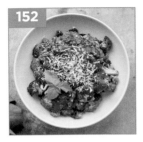
152
B3 Bowl

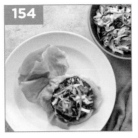
154
BBQ Burgers with Spicy Slaw

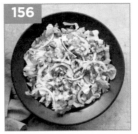
156
BBQ Chicken Salad

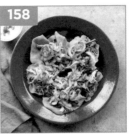
158
BBQ Pulled Pork Tacos with Spicy Slaw

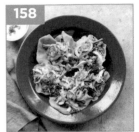
158
Slow Cooker BBQ Pulled Pork

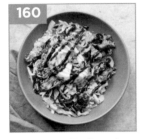
160
BBQ Pulled Pork Buddha Bowl

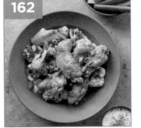
162
Buffalo Cauliflower & Chicken Wings

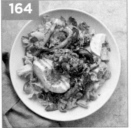
164
Chicken Fajita Salad

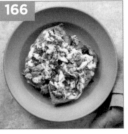
166
Ranch Chicken & Bacon Stuffed Potatoes

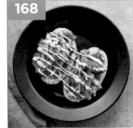
168
Cheesesteak Stuffed Potatoes

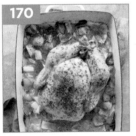
170
Diane's Simple Roast Chicken

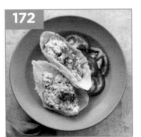
172
Smoky Chicken Salad Lettuce Boats

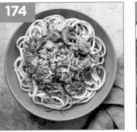
174
Creamy Mustard Chicken with Zoodles

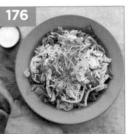
176
Tangy Chicken Salad

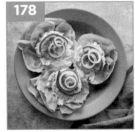
178
Deli Tuna Sliders

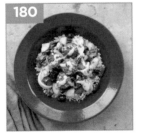
180
Mediterranean Meatball Bowl

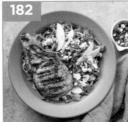
182
Grilled Pork Fall Salad

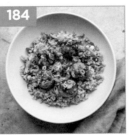
184
Super Garlic Meatballs with Fried Rice

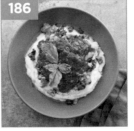
186
Sausage & Spinach "Polenta" Bowl

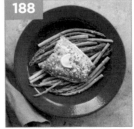
188
Super Garlic Salmon & Vegetables

SNACKS & **SIDES**

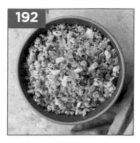
192
Simple Fried Rice

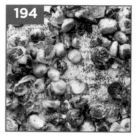
194
Crispy Brussels Sprouts

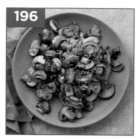
196
Garlic Butter Sautéed Mushrooms

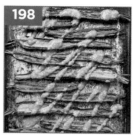
198
Pesto Roasted Carrots

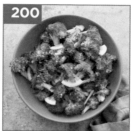
200
Crispy Broccoli

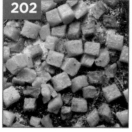
202
Roasted Butternut Squash

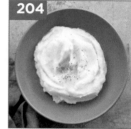
204
Roasted Garlic Cauliflower Polenta

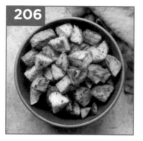
206
Ranch Roasted Potatoes

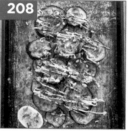
208
Roasted Eggplant Steaks with Tahini Sauce

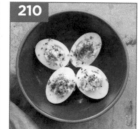
210
Simple Deviled Eggs

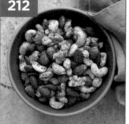
212
Smoky Toasted Nut Mix

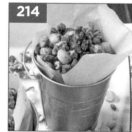
214
Cinnilla Nut Mix

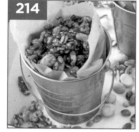
214
Spicy Thai Nut Mix

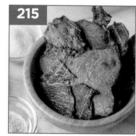
215
Simple Beef Jerky

NOT-SWEET **TREATS**

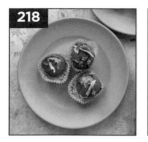
Two-Bite Chocolate
Cream Pies

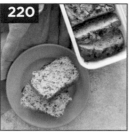
21DSD Cinnamon
Banana Bread

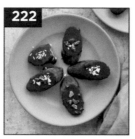
21DSD Frozen
Coco-Monkey Bites

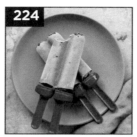
21DSD Fudge Pops

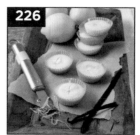
Lemon Vanilla
Meltaways

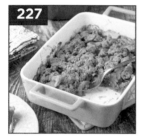
Granny Smith
Apple Crumble

SAUCES, DRESSINGS & **BASICS**

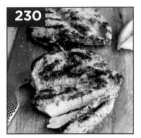
230
Perfectly Grilled
Chicken Breast

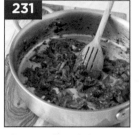
231
Caramelized Onions

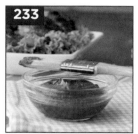
232
21DSD Ketchup

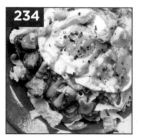
233
21DSD BBQ Sauce

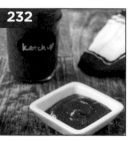
234
Peanut Sauce

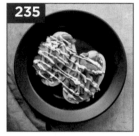
235
Cashew "Cheese"
Sauce

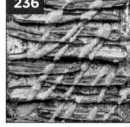
236
Pesto Sauce

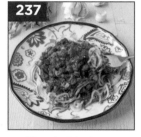
237
Simple Marinara

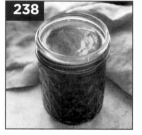
238
Balsamic Vinaigrette
Dressing

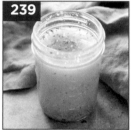
239
Lemon-Herb
Dressing

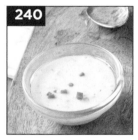
240
Ranch Dressing

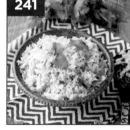
241
Basic Cilantro
Cauli-Rice

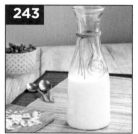
242
Almond Milk & Meal

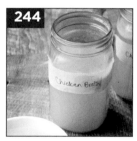
243
Coconut Milk & Flour

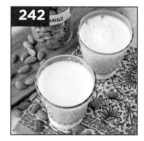
244
Bone Broth

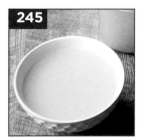
245
Vegetable Broth

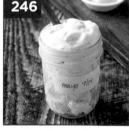
246
Healthy Homemade
Mayonnaise

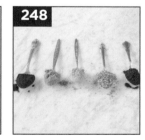
247
Clarified Butter &
Ghee

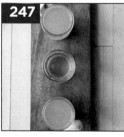
248
Spice Blends

REFERENCES

Ahmed, Serge H., Karine Guillem, and Youna Vandaele. "Sugar Addiction: Pushing the Drug-Sugar Analogy to the Limit." *Current Opinion in Clinical Nutrition and Metabolic Care* 16, no. 4 (July 2013): 434–439.

Aitken, Tara J., Venuz Y. Greenfield, and Kate M. Wassum. "Nucleus Accumbens Core Dopamine Signaling Tracks the Need-Based Motivational Value of Food-Paired Cues." *Journal of Neurochemistry* 136, no. 5 (March 2016): 1026–1036.

Bargh, John A. "The Four Horsemen of Automaticity: Awareness, Intention, Efficiency, and Control in Social Cognition." In *Handbook of Social Cognition*, 2nd ed., edited by Robert S. Wyer Jr. and Thomas K. Srull, 1–40. New York: Psychology Press, 2014.

Beeler, Jeff A., James E. McCutcheon, Zhen F. H. Cao, Mari Murakami, Erin Alexander, Mitchell F. Roitman, and Xiaoxi Zhuang. "Taste Uncoupled from Nutrition Fails to Sustain the Reinforcing Properties of Food." *European Journal of Neuroscience* 36, no. 4 (August 2012): 2533–2546.

Bello, Nicholas T., and Andras Hajnal. "Dopamine and Binge Eating Behaviors." *Pharmacology, Biochemistry and Behavior* 97 (2010): 25–33.

Brown, Holden T., James E. McCutcheon, Jackson J. Cone, Michael E. Ragozzino, and Mitchell F. Roitman. "Primary Food Reward and Reward-Predictive Stimuli Evoke Different Patterns of Phasic Dopamine Signaling Throughout the Striatum." *European Journal of Neuroscience* 34, no. 12 (December 2011): 1997–2006.

Caravaggio, Fernando, Carol Borlido, Margaret Hahn, Zhe Feng, Gagan Fervaha, Philip Gerretsen, Shinichiro Nakajima, et al. "Reduced Insulin Sensitivity Is Related to Less Endogenous Dopamine at D2/3 Receptors in the Ventral Striatum of Healthy Nonobese Humans." *International Journal of Neuropsychopharmacology* 18, no. 7 (May 2015).

Cone, Jackson J., James E. McCutcheon, and Mitchell F. Roitman. "Ghrelin Acts as an Interface between Physiological State and Phasic Dopamine Signaling." *Journal of Neuroscience* 34, no. 14 (April 2014): 4905–4913.

Gardner, Benjamin, Gert-Jan de Bruijn, and Phillippa Lally. "A Systematic Review and Meta-analysis of Applications of the Self-Report Habit Index to Nutrition and Physical Activity Behaviours." *Annals of Behavioral Medicine* 42, no. 2 (October 2011): 174–187.

Gardner, Benjamin, Phillippa Lally, and Jane Wardle. "Making Health Habitual: The Psychology of 'Habit-Formation' and General Practice." *British Journal of General Practice* 62, no. 205 (December 2012): 664–666.

Han, Wenfei, Luis A. Tellez, Jingjing Niu, Gary J. Schwartz, Anthony van den Pol, Ivan E. de Araujo, et al. "Striatal Dopamine Links Gastrointestinal Rerouting to Altered Sweet Appetite." *Cell Metabolism* 23 (January 2016): 1–10.

Lally, P., A. Chipperfield, and J. Wardle. "Healthy Habits: Efficacy of Simple Advice on Weight Control Based on a Habit-Formation Model." *International Journal of Obesity* 32 (2008): 700–707.

Lally, Phillippa, Cornelia H. M. Van Jaarsveld, Henry W. W. Potts, and Jane Wardle. "How Are Habits Formed: Modelling Habit Formation in the Real World." *European Journal of Social Psychology* 40 (2010): 998–1009.

Lally, Phillippa, Jane Wardle, and Benjamin Gardner. "Experiences of Habit Formation: A Qualitative Study." *Psychology, Health & Medicine* 16, no. 4 (2011): 484–489.

Lally, Phillippa, Naomi Bartle, and Jane Wardle. "Social Norms and Diet in Adolescents." *Appetite* 57 (2011): 623–627.

Lally, Phillippa, Lucy Cooke, Laura McGowan, Helen Croker, Naomi Bartle, and Jane Wardle. "Parents' Misperceptions of Social Norms for Pre-school Children's Snacking Behaviour." *Public Health Nutrition* 15, no. 9 (2012): 1678–1682.

Mitra, Anaya, Blake A. Gosnell, Helgi B. Schiöth, Martha K. Grace, Anica Klockars, Pawel K. Olszewski, and Allen S. Levine. "Chronic Sugar Intake Dampens Feeding-Related Activity of Neurons Synthesizing a Satiety Mediator, Oxytocin." *Peptides* 31 (2010): 1346–1352.

Roemer, Ewald, Matthias K. Schorp, Jean-Jacques Piadé, Jeffrey I. Seeman, Donald E. Leyden, and Hans-Juergen Haussmann. "Scientific Assessment of the Use of Sugars as Cigarette Tobacco Ingredients: A Review of Published and Other Publicly Available Studies." *Critical Reviews in Toxicology* 42, no. 3 (2012): 244–278.

Schulte, Erica M., Nicole M. Avena, and Ashley N. Gearhardt. "Which Foods May Be Addictive? The Roles of Processing, Fat Content, and Glycemic Load." *PLOS One*, February 18, 2015, https://doi.org/10.1371/journal.pone.0117959.

Shnitko, Tatiana A., and Donita L. Robinson. "Regional Variation in Phasic Dopamine Release during Alcohol and Sucrose Self-Administration in Rats." *ACS Chemical Neuroscience* 6, no. 1 (2015): 147–154.

Tellez, Luis A., Xueying Ren, Wenfei Han, Sara Medina, Jozélia G. Ferreira, Catherine W. Yeckel, and Ivan E. de Araujo. "Glucose Utilization Rates Regulate Intake Levels of Artificial Sweeteners." *Journal of Physiology* 591, no. 22 (November 2013): 5727–5744.

Tellez, Luis A., Wenfei Han, Xiaobing Zhang, Tatiana L. Ferreira, Isaac O. Perez, Sara J. Shammah-Lagnado, Anthony N. van den Pol, et al. "Separate Circuitries Encode the Hedonic and Nutritional Values of Sugar." *Nature Neuroscience* 19 (2016): 465–470.

Ustione, Alessandro, and David W. Piston. "Dopamine Synthesis and D3 Receptor Activation in Pancreatic ß-Cells Regulates Insulin Secretion and Intracellular [Ca2+] Oscillations." *Molecular Endocrinology* 26, no. 11 (November 2012): 1928–1940.

Wegner, Daniel M., and John A. Bargh. "Control and Automaticity in Social Life." In *Handbook of Social Psychology*, 4th ed., vol 1., edited by Daniel T. Gilbert, Susan T. Fiske, and Gardner Lindzey, 446–496. New York: McGraw-Hill, 1998.

Westwater, Margaret L., Paul C. Fletcher, and Hisham Ziauddeen. "Sugar Addiction: The State of the Science." *European Journal of Nutrition* 55, suppl. 2 (November 2016): 55–69.

DAILY LESSON INDEX

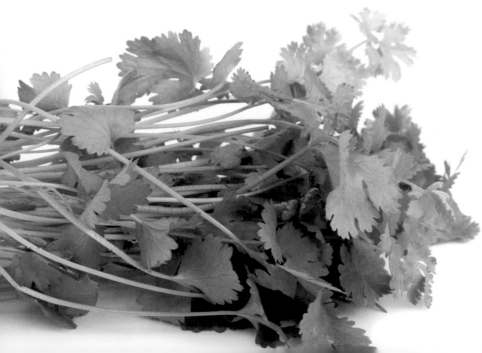

POST-DETOX WEEK

INDEX

GRATITUDE

As I complete what is effectively my sixth publication, I always take a few moments to think about what drives me and keeps me going when it gets tough to work on a new book.

You, the reader, are at the forefront of my mind throughout this entire process. As I conceptualized this book over the last few years, met you in person at events, talked to you while you completed your program, and interacted with you via social media, your faces and your stories have motivated me. Perhaps it seems obvious to say that I write books for you, but it's true. This process is extremely difficult for me: as many of you know, I'm something of a "rebel," and I constantly need that guiding light—the vision of you at home using the books I write in your everyday life—to push me through each part of the process. I thank you all, not only for buying my books and sharing them with your friends and families but also for engaging with me and for using my work to change your life for the better— beginning with what you eat, but ever expanding into other areas of your life, which I truly do hope to reach. My goal is always to help you live a happier, more fulfilling life, so if becoming healthier is the first step, let it be just that—the first step. I hope to be here to encourage you along far more steps as time goes on, and I appreciate your presence.

Team Balanced Bites, as a whole, collectively: You are my work family, and I love the opportunity to lead you all to achieving things together that none of us would be able to achieve apart.

Niki: Who'd have known that an email shot-in-the-dark would evolve into such a close working relationship that's not only productive but also fun and filled with creative ideas?! I'm honestly not sure how I would have gotten through the recipe process without you, nor am I sure I'd have actually committed to writing this book without knowing you'd be here alongside me through the process. You stepped up in ways I didn't expect, and I was so proud to let you run with your work and contributions to the recipes and meal plan. Our readers are the ones who will truly benefit from your work, and I hope you feel immense joy and gratification knowing that. Gold star!

Holly: You may have introduced yourself with dark chocolate all those years ago, but your constant presence on this team has been an absolute anchor to the work we've all done together for so long. Knowing I was able to trust your leadership with our 21DSD Coaches—and throughout all of our programs—has been a true joy. Your compassion and empathy, not only for other practitioners but also for participants in our programs, are true gifts, and I thank you for sharing them with me, our team, and our community.

April: You're a rock in our community, supporting our participants every day as they step along their journey. Thank you for unwaveringly providing your attention to their needs year after year. I know many of our community members have been touched by you and your presence—and by all of the #coffeewithfosterdogs you've posted year after year!

Lindsey: You're the lighthouse that guides not only me but our entire team. I have my crazy ideas, but you help me harness the creativity and get it onto the calendar so it'll happen. I value the solutions and contributions you've made to our team for so many years and the sass, counterpoints, and direct feedback you're not afraid to serve up. Thanks for being a badass and for pushing me to deliver on my own dreams.

Moriah: You're a different person than you were just a couple of years ago when you first joined this team. I'm so proud of how independent you've become in your work and design direction, and I'm so grateful to rely on you to execute my visions—and to contribute yours to them to make them better. This book began as a vision of mine, was amplified by the team's ideas, and was brought to life on paper at your hands. We're so lucky to have you on this team.

Kate: When you joined the team, we needed some major organizational glue, and you swooped in to straight-up handle it! I'm so grateful for your reliably complete and detailed work on every project you touch. In fact, when you finish things I didn't even ask for ahead of time, I'm consistently amazed and impressed. I can't wait to see what we create as time goes on with you on the team—I'm so grateful for your presence.

Amanda: You've supported the creative execution of video content for our team with skill and grace. I'm so excited to see where your work takes things and how much it continues to amplify our online program in the coming years. You continually strive to improve and push yourself to learn new ways of doing things, and it shows in each new video you create. You've been a gift to our team.

Moderators: For your community support over the years, I am truly grateful. I know our participants rely on your guidance and speedy answers to their questions and they appreciate you as much as I do!

Coaches: For the last several years, I've had the great honor of guiding and leading you all as you've developed into amazing representatives of this program. I'm so proud of what you all do to reach those near you and far from you. I'm continually impressed by the work you do and how you take this message of health into your communities in creative ways. You help so many people who need this information, and I'm grateful that you've put your trust in me and this team to support you in your efforts. I hope this book serves as another amazing tool for your work and that your participants love it.

Scott: Thank you for being my rock, for dealing with my photography studio taking over the living room in our new home, and for getting me kombucha and making dinners while this book was being finished up.

And, lastly, to the team at Victory Belt, as always: Thanks for trusting my ideas and for allowing my visions to come to life despite my unconventional process. Erin, it's always a pleasure to have you on my side for what proves to be the most painful part of the entire process (and for that, I'm sorry). Susan, thanks for pushing to help make the tour happen at a tough time of year. And Erich, thanks for being not only a supportive publisher but also a friend and a mentor. I'm truly grateful for the opportunity to be published.